The Situational Judgement Test at a Glance

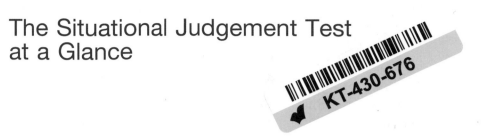

This title is also available as an e-book.
For more details, please see
www.wiley.com/buy/9781118490983
or scan this QR code:

The Situational Judgement Test at a Glance

Frances Varian

Frances Varian is a final year medical student at Warwick University and was seconded by Warwick Medical School to help develop situational judgement educational material and practice questions designed to enhance students' non-technical skills.

Lara Cartwright

Lara Cartwright is Senior Careers Consultant at Warwick Medical School and a member of the Association of Graduate Careers Advisory Services (AGCAS) and the Medical Careers Advisor's Network (MCAN).

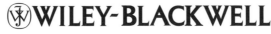

WILEY-BLACKWELL

A John Wiley & Sons, Ltd., Publication

Registered office: John Wiley & Sons, Ltd, The Atrium, Southern Gate, Chichester, West Sussex, PO19 8SQ, UK

Editorial offices: 9600 Garsington Road, Oxford, OX4 2DQ, UK
The Atrium, Southern Gate, Chichester, West Sussex, PO19 8SQ, UK
111 River Street, Hoboken, NJ 07030-5774, USA

For details of our global editorial offices, for customer services and for information about how to apply for permission to reuse the copyright material in this book please see our website at www.wiley.com/wiley-blackwell.

Library of Congress Cataloging-in-Publication Data
Varian, Frances.
   The situational judgement test at a glance / Frances Varian, Lara Cartwright.
       p. ; cm.
   Includes bibliographical references and index.
   ISBN 978-1-118-49098-3 (pbk. : alk. paper)
   I. Cartwright, Lara.   II. Title.
   [DNLM: 1. Decision Making–Great Britain–Case Reports.   2. Decision Making–Great Britain–Examination Questions.   3. Professional Practice–Great Britain–Case Reports.
4. Professional Practice–Great Britain–Examination Questions.   5. Behavior–Great Britain–Case Reports.   6. Behavior–Great Britain–Examination Questions.   7. Judgment–Great Britain–Case Reports.   8. Judgment–Great Britain–Examination Questions.
9. Psychological Tests–Great Britain.   10. Test Taking Skills–Great Britain.
W 18.2]

   150.28'7–dc23

                                        2012031981

A catalogue record for this book is available from the British Library.

Wiley also publishes its books in a variety of electronic formats. Some content that appears in printmay not be available in electronic books.

Cover image: Bigstock © Michael Jung
Cover design by Meaden Creative

Set in 10/12.5 pt Times by Toppan Best-set Premedia Limited

1   2013

Contents

Preface

What are Situational Judgement Tests?

Exactly what they say on the tin! A way of assessing how you judge a situation encountered within the workplace. They are not designed to test your clinical knowledge and skills; they are designed to test your attitudes and ethical values. With this in mind, the ISFP (Improving Selection to Foundation Programme) developed nine domains of assessment for UKFPO (United Kingdom Foundation Programme Office) application:

- Commitment to Professionalism
- Learning and Professional Development
- Working Effectively as Part of a Team
- Patient Focus
- Problem Solving and Decision-Making
- Self-Awareness and Insight
- Coping with Pressure
- Organisation and Planning
- Effective Communication

These are assessed in two ways: either by ranking five responses from most appropriate to least appropriate, or by selecting the three most appropriate responses to the situation in question. The response is then evaluated against a predetermined scoring key decided by the subject-matter experts. Download the SJT Monograph on the UKFPO website www.foundationprogramme.nhs.uk for more information. All scenarios are evaluated by doctors in terms of their applicability to real life. The SJT scenarios in this book have also been scrutinised and cover similar issues to those offered in the 2010 pilot (AMRC 2010) as well as real situations submitted by foundation year interviewees. The following chapters deal with the nine areas above and detail juniors' experiences from their time on the wards:

1. **Introduction:** this chapter includes how best to prepare for the SJT, some handy ways of handling the scenarios, as well as some things to look out for on the wards. It also evaluates the importance of self-awareness and insight with respect to conducting yourself day to day in clinical practice.

2. **Professionalism**: this chapter covers the behaviours expected of a junior doctor together with codes of conduct, including issues of confidentiality.

3. **Pressures and prioritisation**: this chapter focuses on the common pressures of an FY1: probity, ward rounds, discharges, prescribing and consenting. It also addresses learning and professional development, managing career progression as well as what to do if your job requires considerable juggling. Finally, this chapter considers prioritisation – including bleep etiquette – in which organisation and planning are integral.

4. **Communication**: this chapter engages with common pitfalls connected with record-keeping and tips for successful documentation. Also covered are communication difficulties involving translators, disabilities and relatives.

5. **Patient focus**: this chapter deals with how to be the best doctor for your patients, detailing responsibility for patient advocacy, capacity, end of life care and problem-solving with respect to handling difficult patients.

6. **Effective teamwork**: this chapter outlines effective handovers, handling professional – and personal – conflicts and understanding others' roles so you can most effectively work as a team-player. These include the roles of nursing, radiology and laboratory staff as well as those more involved in your social support such as educational supervisors and foundation directors.

7. **SJT practice material**: this chapter covers a method of approaching an SJT question and contains 50 practice SJT questions. It concludes with a way of creating your own examples and gives tips on how to develop your own learning on the wards.

The aim here is to get you thinking of ways to approach the SJT under exam conditions, as well as to enhance your understanding of the role expected of you as an FY1. The approach to this text replicated that of the ISFP; interviewing doctors, patients and healthcare professionals about the expected qualities of a junior doctor. This material was then integrated into the FY1 job analysis specifications outlined by the ISFP (Patterson et al 2010) to provide you with a comprehensive guide to tackling the SJTs.

Finally, this material has been reviewed by students who sat the 2011 pilot. They have approved its utility as a preparation for the SJT exam. Please note that, whilst the information closely adheres to GMC guidance, you should refer back to the original documentation for advice in any potentially difficult situation. The information here is designed to assist your learning process in thinking about what you **should** do in a situation, and not what you necessarily **would** do in practice. All the examples are from doctors' real-life experiences working on the wards; from which the SJT practice questions have been adapted. The names have been changed in some cases to protect identities. For accuracy, these questions and explanations have been reviewed by an independent writer for the UKFPO SJT selection paper, senior clinicians and foundation trainees. These questions cannot guarantee success in the SJT, but have been developed and designed to replicate as far as possible the types of scenarios encountered in the formal assessment paper (AMRC 2010).

Frances Varian
Lara Cartwright

Acknowledgements

We would like to thank all those people who gave their time and expertise to advise us in writing this book. We would particularly like to thank the medical students who reviewed the material – especially James Coe, James Webster, Ayrton Goddard, Jennifer Goddard, Graeme Mattison, James Haddock, Adrian Hayes and David Andrews – as well as all the patients who kindly gave their time – and their stories – to help create an interesting read.

Special thanks are due to Katherine Mundy – author of the children's book *Thomas Young and the Go To Tunnel* – for her artistic talent in creating the original illustrations, and to Graeme Chambers for his work in translating them into the Figures in this book.

List of Contributors

Maggie Allen
Consultant Rheumatologist, Associate Medical Director of
Education and Foundation Programme Clinical Tutor
University Hospital Coventry and Warwickshire, Coventry

Nicholas Ashley
Foundation Year 1
West Midlands

Michael Baker
General Practitioner and Educational Supervisor
Solihull

Anthony Blacker
Consultant Urologist
University Hospital Coventry and Warwickshire, Coventry

Lara Cartwright
Senior Careers Consultant
Warwick Medical School
University of Warwick, Coventry

Samyami S. Chowdhury
Foundation Year 2
West Midlands

Linda Crinigan
Clinical Skills Practitioner
University Hospital Coventry and Warwickshire, Coventry

Daniel Higman
Consultant Vascular Surgeon and Foundation Programme Director
Coventry
Warwickshire Foundation School
University Hospital Coventry and Warwickshire, Coventry

Carl Hammond
Foundation Year 2
West Midlands

Fraz Hussain
Foundation Year 2
West Midlands

Colette Marshall
Consultant Vascular Surgeon
University Hospital Coventry and Warwickshire, Coventry

Sarah Sharp
Foundation Year 2
West Midlands

Edward Simmonds
Consultant Paediatrician and Foundation Programme Year 1
Clinical Tutor
University Hospital Coventry and Warwickshire, Coventry

Anne-Marie Slowther
Associate Professor of Clinical Ethics
Warwick Medical School
University of Warwick, Coventry

Jacqueline Timeyin
Specialist Trainee, Year 1, Paediatrics
Manchester

Desmond Varian
Psychiatric Nurse
Cumbria

Frances Varian
Final year Medical Student, Graduate-Entry Programme
Warwick Medical School
University of Warwick, Coventry

Marakatham Venkataraman
Consultant Paediatrician and Foundation Programme Clinical
Lead
George Eliot Hospital, Nuneaton

Ayman Zaghloul
Consultant Psychiatrist
Caludon Centre, Walsgrave, Coventry

List of Abbreviations

ABG	Arterial Blood Gas		**IMCA**	Independent Mental Capacity Advocate
BMA	British Medical Association		**INR**	International Normalised Ratio
BNF	British National Formulary		**ISFP**	Improving Selection to the Foundation Programme
BSL	British Sign Language		**ITU**	Intensive Treatment Unit
CAB	Citizens Advice Bureau		**KMR**	Kohner Medical Record
CAE	Clinically Adverse Event		**MCA**	Mental Capacity Act
CRP	C-Reactive Protein		**MEWS**	Modified Early Warning Score
CS	Caesarean Section		**MHA**	Mental Health Act
CT	Computerised Tomography		**MHRA**	Medicine and Healthcare products Regulatory Agency
DDA	Disability Discrimination Act		**MPS**	Medical Protection Society
DH	Department of Health		**MST**	Morphine Sulphate Tablets
DKA	Diabetic Ketoacidosis		**NKDA**	No Known Drug Allergies
DNAR	Do Not Attempt Resuscitation		**OT**	Occupational Therapist
DVLA	Driver and Vehicle Licensing Agency		**OTC**	Over-The-Counter
EHRC	Equality Human Rights Commission		**PALS**	Patient Advice and Liaison Service
EOL	End of Life		**PRN**	Pro Re Nata
ESR	Erythrocyte Sedimentation Rate		**QOL**	Quality of Life
FTP	Fitness to Practise		**RCP**	Royal College of Physicians
FY1	Foundation Year 1		**SBAR**	Situation Background Assessment Recommendation
FY2	Foundation Year 2		**SHO**	Senior House Officer
GMC	General Medical Council		**SJT**	Situational Judgement Tests
GP	General Practitioner		**ST1**	Specialist Training Year 1
GUM	Genito-Urinary Medicine		**STAT**	*Statim* (immediately)
HLC	Hospital Liaison Committee		**STI**	Sexually Transmitted Infection
ICE	Ideas Concerns and Expectations		**UKFPO**	United Kingdom Foundation Programme Office

1 Introduction

Mike, GP *"Recognise where your personality is and try to understand what you are like and how you get job satisfaction; in the end work in that area . . . you'll feel like you're under far less pressure if you do that"*

This book lends insight into the kinds of scenario that a foundation doctor encounters. However, before we dive in to discuss life on the wards, let's take some time to consider your unique approach to the role of an FY1. SJT questions require you to think about what you **should** do, i.e. how to handle a situation most appropriately. First though, consider what you most likely **would** do. Gaining insight into this discrepancy will be helpful in approaching the SJT and, more importantly, in continuing your professional development.

Considering what you most likely **would** do requires an understanding of your own characteristics and behaviour. This helps you to:
- Work with colleagues who might behave differently to you.
- Communicate effectively with team members, patients and their families.
- Evaluate your response to working under pressure.
- Work out how to best define your priorities.
- Interpret feedback in relation to your performance.
- Monitor your well-being at work.
- Perform your best in selection processes: from the SJT through to specialty training.

Personality

People behave in different ways, depending on the circumstances or the people they are with. However, it is widely accepted that some aspects of personality stay stable and, over the years, personality testing has evolved to measure these domains. You do not have to take a formal personality test, but understanding a little about personality theory can help you to understand yourself in relation to the role of an FY1. There are five widely recognised domains along which personality is measured, known as "the Big Five". These are shown in Figure 1.1.

It is helpful to see each of the "big five" as a continuum, with most people coming out somewhere in the middle rather than being able to be labelled as one thing or another. Research has shown that domains are relevant across cultural boundaries (McCrae et al. 2005).

Openness and neuroticism can be used as examples to show how people respond differently to taking a test like the SJT. If you think you are on the high side of the neurotic scale, and the thought of the SJT stresses you out, you may find the wealth of practice material in this book invaluable in calming your nerves. If you are more of a conformist on the openness scale, you might find the checklists of good practice and procedures to your liking.

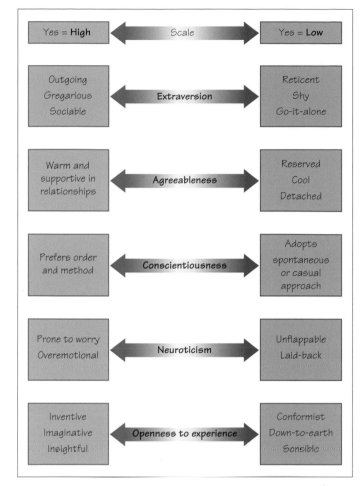

Figure 1.1 The "Big Five"

Different personality types can do the same job equally well. They just bring their own unique stamp to the way they do it. However, different personality traits can result in different individual experiences and challenges in relation to the same job. Here are some examples with respect to the domains covered by the SJT.

Professionalism
- If you are high on the extraversion scale, you might find it more difficult to rein yourself in on social networking sites and resist talking in an unguarded way.
- Conversely, if you are low on this scale, you might find it harder to challenge the actions of others and speak out when you see bad practice.
- If you are highly conscientious, you might find it easier to maintain punctuality.
- If you are highly neurotic, you might find it particularly hard to switch off from stressful days.

The Situational Judgement Test at a Glance, First Edition. Frances Varian and Lara Cartwright.
© 2013 John Wiley & Sons, Ltd. Published 2013 by John Wiley & Sons, Ltd.

Pressures and prioritisation

• Being highly conscientious and only mildly neurotic will make it easier to work under pressure and remain calm and in control.

• If you are highly open to new experiences, you will have an advantage when it comes to managing rapidly changing situations.

• Conversely, when following protocols, being low on openness may stand you in good stead.

• If you are high in agreeableness you may tend to seek help from others naturally; a key factor in some of the SJT questions.

Effective communication and patient focus

• Introverts may find relating to patients' concerns a more difficult aspect of the FY1 role.

• If you are highly neurotic you must remember not to relay your anxieties to the patient; having confidence in your skills as a doctor is an important aspect of the doctor–patient relationship.

• Being highly agreeable lends itself to good communication with relatives; if you are at the other end of the scale, you may have to work harder to empathise with others.

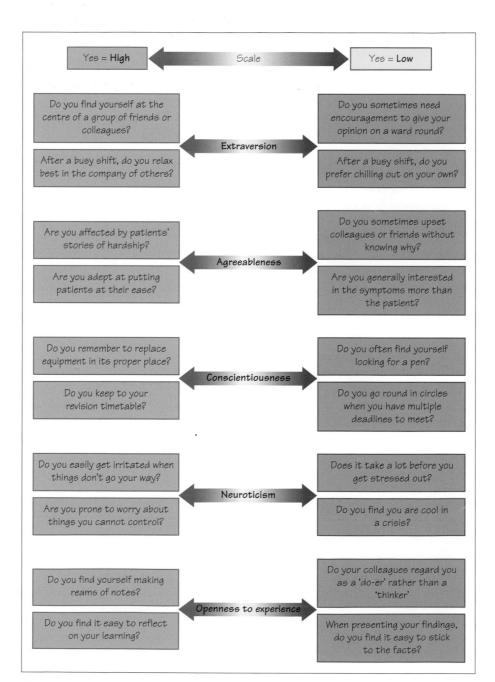

Figure 1.2 Understanding yourself

Teamwork

• If you tend to "think outside the box" when problems occur, your openness to experience may puzzle or even frustrate your more cautious colleagues.

• If you are high in agreeableness, you may find your priority is to promote harmony within your team. This may also mean that you find it more difficult to challenge colleagues who do not pull their weight.

• Being high in conscientiousness will be appreciated by your colleagues

Teamwork is so fundamental to the FY1 role; it is examined in more depth in Chapter 6.

How is this relevant?

Bear in mind the different personality traits when you test yourself during the course of this book, especially when you compare what you **would** do to what you **should** do (i.e. the right answer). When there are discrepancies, ask yourself why they exist. Is it, for example, because you don't like asking for help? Reflect on your personality and behaviour and consider how you could improve your performance. This is an important skill which will prove fruitful to your future development as a doctor. Finally, it is important that you seek out feedback on your non-technical skills in addition to your clinical competencies throughout your clinical attachments. This is part and parcel of continuing professional growth.

The questions in Figure 1.2 will help to guide you towards one side of a particular trait or the other. Although Figure 1.2 does not constitute a formal personality test, if you answer "yes" easily to one set of prompts, it will give you an indication of which end of the scale you gravitate towards. If you wish for a more formal assessment, most commercially available personality tests include some measurement of these domains. Consequently, you may find it useful to complete an online personality questionnaire such as the Myers-Briggs Type Inventory (Myers and Briggs Foundation n.d.).

2 Professionalism

Mithun, Consultant Psychiatrist *"Take pride in being a professional . . . there are only a few professions which carry such a lot of trust and responsibility. People come to you at times of their weakness, not at their strength: you have to be trustworthy. Medical knowledge is only part of treatment: people skills, the instillation of hope, your smile, bedside manners . . . all those skills are so important. At the end of the day doctors are tools – we have knowledge and apply solutions scientifically – it's how we relay those to the patient that is of the greatest importance."*

In terms of professionalism, foundation doctors are expected to:
- Display integrity, honesty and trustworthiness.
- Understand the role of being a doctor, including ethical responsibilities and respect for confidentiality.
- Be punctual and reliable.
- Own up to mistakes.
- Challenge actions and knowledge which may put others at risk.

What is integrity?

Integrity is mentioned in connection with the healthcare profession in many situations, but few people consider why. Integrity is about being honest and upholding moral principles – always. This is important to realise, because you cannot simply put on your professional face at work and let loose as soon as you exit the hospital doors. As a doctor, you must have integrity woven into every aspect of your life. You are a public figure and must therefore meet public expectations for the security of the profession.

Ultimately, you have to be honest, trustworthy and respectable in both your work and your personal life. This leads onto the next discussion: social networking. Social networking is a common area where doctors and medical students can get caught out.

Social networking

As highlighted, professionalism as a doctor should extend through every aspect of your life. Doctors are expected to behave like doctors. Say, for example, your friend decides to upload a photo of you looking drunk and dishevelled on a Friday night; this might not appear so hilarious to a patient who decides to Google you. Unprofessional behaviour online will impact on your integrity, because social media has increasingly blurred the distinction between our personal and professional lives.

THE BMA (2011) RECOMMENDS THE FOLLOWING:

- Be conscious that your online image will impact on your professionalism.
- Posting about patients or colleagues however informal and "confidential" is inappropriate – think about how that will reflect on you as a person.
- Sort out your privacy settings to protect personal information.
- Politely refuse friend requests from current or former patients and explain to the patient the reasons why it would be inappropriate for you to accept.
- Your ethical and legal duty to protect patient confidentiality is the same on the internet as anywhere else.

Always consider whether the information you present online could challenge public confidence in the medical profession. Moreover, consider whether it could change your reputation with colleagues at work.

Chris, Consultant *"I don't mind Facebook, I am friends with my colleagues and aware of that fact . . . . I never post anything other than the mundane to protect myself as a professional. Sometimes people forget who they are friends with. I experienced a situation where two secretaries were publically bullying another online and being extremely derogatory. I had to discipline them for it as that kind of behaviour wouldn't be acceptable in the office and certainly not online".*

The Department of Health (DH 2010) devised six principles by which patient-identifiable information should be utilised:
1. **Justified** – what is the purpose of sharing the information?
2. **Necessary** – how will sharing this information benefit the patient?
3. **Minimum** – only share what needs to be shared. For example, if you are referring a patient with a broken wrist for physiotherapy, you don't need to tell the physio that they also are being treated for chlamydia. Be responsible and think about what you share.
4. **Need-to-know basis** – as above, make sure you tell them what they need to know and nothing more.
5. **Be aware of your role** – you are their doctor, respect the fact that patients trust you and be aware that you have a duty to uphold that confidence in the public eye. Doctors without trust are like buckets with a hole in: not very good at all!
6. **Legal** – if you are unsure of a boundary, always check it with a senior before you share anything.

The Situational Judgement Test at a Glance, First Edition. Frances Varian and Lara Cartwright.

14 © 2013 John Wiley & Sons, Ltd. Published 2013 by John Wiley & Sons, Ltd.

Understanding confidentiality

There is a wealth of information regarding confidentiality and generally it is very well taught at medical school. Basically, you need to understand the principles of information-sharing, and, if you know those, you should know what to do regardless of the scenario.

If you are unsure, always seek advice from a senior colleague in the first instance. Any scenario where confidentiality could potentially be compromised should not be rushed. Beyond this, there are assigned figures within the NHS known as Caldicott guardians. These are typically board-level clinicians who resolve local issues regarding information-sharing that go beyond the level of a senior colleague. Typical situations in which Caldicott guardians become involved include (DH 2010):

- police requesting information
- a patient requesting for their records to be deleted
- serious confidentiality breaches

It is enough simply to know about the existence of these figures. You should get in touch with your foundation programme clinical lead or foundation programme co-ordinator for all concerns involving the legal department. FY1s are not in a position to handle such matters, nor are they expected to do so.

What should you do if confidentiality is breached?

A breach of confidentiality is not something that can be 'undone' and puts a serious question mark over your professional conduct. If a patient feels confidentiality has been breached, they can action a disciplinary via the GMC which has serious consequences for your career (Ministry of Ethics 2010). However, rarely does a patient decide to prosecute for a confidentiality breach. If something does happen, the Medical Protection Society (MPS 2010) argues you can best handle this by:

1. Establishing what happened and what went wrong.
2. Offering the patient an explanation and an apology.
3. Giving assurance that lessons have been learned.
4. Identifying how mistakes can be avoided in the future.

Common situations where confidentiality is breached are (MPS 2011):

- In a lift or canteen.
- In A&E departments and on wards where parents and relatives are in close proximity.
- Through patient's notes: commonly left in places where they are easily accessed by the public.
- Through computers, faxes and printers: information becomes easily visible.
- In pubs and restaurants (see Figure 2.1).

These two examples illustrate accidental breaches of confidentiality. Key learning points from these involve taking particular care with relatives and being sensitive, but recognising that your responsibilities are to the patient first and foremost.

Ashleigh, FY1 *"I have a really loud carrying voice. One incident that stays with me involved a lady on the respiratory ward who was dying. Her relatives were down the corridor. I was discussing the patient with the consultant behind the curtain on the ward round and we were saying how she was going to die soon. Afterwards the family approached me – they didn't complain or anything – but repeated what was said behind the curtain: 'so you think that she is going to die soon, do you?' It was obvious they had heard us . . . . I apologised profusely, as I didn't mean for them to hear what we were saying. Whilst our conversation wasn't insensitive, it's not nice to hear your relatives are going to die in such frank terms. It was pretty horrible . . . . I always dial down the volume now!"*

Jack, ST1 *"There was an 80-year-old gentleman who had a haemorrhagic stroke secondary to brain metastasis. He wasn't known to have cancer. The family came to speak to the registrar who then made the mistake of telling the family about it before the patient knew. The family then said they didn't want the patient to know. So the registrar listened to this and didn't tell him! When the consultant found out, he was very angry and went straight to tell the patient what had happened. His theory was – quite rightly – if the patient found out and didn't want the family to know then that ship had sailed. The patient has the right not to let the family know: not the other way round. In the end it was all OK, the patient was fine with the family knowing, but it shouldn't have happened."*

Information-sharing and confidentiality can be a bit of a minefield, especially at first when everything is so new. Described below are a few scenarios to be familiar with. Remember, though, that every trust should have local policy guidelines on these matters, and, if you are ever unsure, always seek senior advice.

The DVLA

What should you do if you think a patient is not fit to drive?

The Driver and Vehicle Licensing Agency (DVLA) are responsible for road safety and have strict guidance on health conditions and fitness to drive. Three things to note are:

1. It is the driver's legal responsibility to notify the DVLA.
2. You are responsible for telling the patient that their condition may affect their driving (see Figure 2.2).
3. Document in the notes what you have told them.

Some common conditions that **patients** will need to notify to the DVLA are:

- Epilepsy or a seizure.
- Diabetes mellitus on any treatment that can cause hypoglycaemia.
- Acute psychosis.
- Severe mood disorders or neuroses: especially if they may attempt suicide at the wheel.

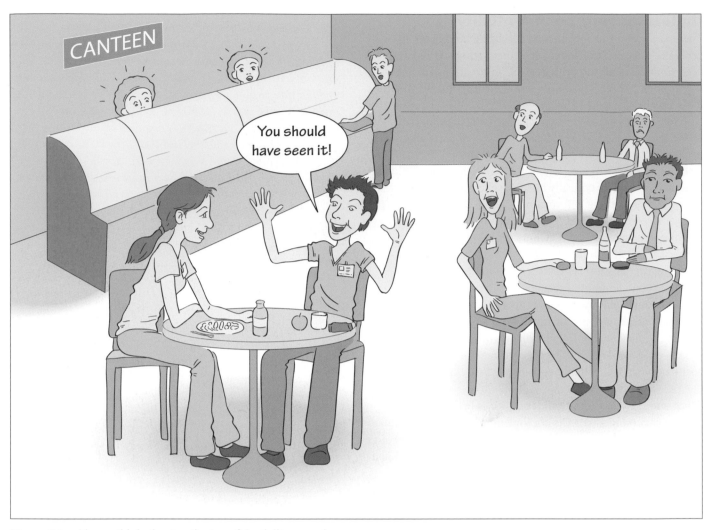

Figure 2.1 Always think about patient confidentiality . . . wherever you are

• Alcohol and drug abuse: especially if you suspect they may drive whilst intoxicated.

Some common conditions where you would advise a period of time off from driving, but they don't need to formally notify the DVLA are:
• Stroke/TIA
• Acute Coronary Syndromes (ACS)

The criteria for those with "group 2 entitlement", i.e. lorry drivers, differ from this. Make sure you enquire about occupation so that the patient has the correct information.

If you are unsure what to do, your options are to (GMC 2009b):
1. Seek advice from a senior colleague.
2. Consult your local policy document or the DVLA (2011) *"At a glance guide to the current medical standards of fitness to drive"*. Here you should get the information you require about a variety of disorders and conditions that can impair a patient's fitness to drive.
3. Seek advice from the DVLA or their medical advisor; probably not your first port of call as this will take time.

What happens if your patient disagrees with you?
Advise them to seek a second medical opinion but not to drive in the meantime.

What happens if they ignore you and carry on driving anyway?
• Educate them about the consequences of driving against medical advice to try and stop them; but be reasonable – you cannot use force.
• Use persuasion of friends and relatives if appropriate.

What happens if that fails?
THEN you are advised to notify the DVLA – but tell the patient that you are going to do this first.

Patients involved in serious crime

You are in A&E and you are notified that a patient is coming in with a stabbing injury, what should you do?
Obviously your A to E approach and acute medical assessment come first, but you need to take account of the following:

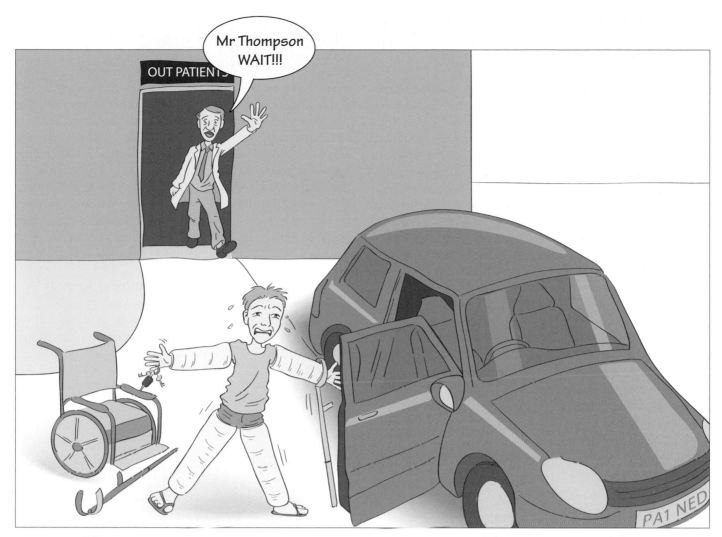

Figure 2.2 Tell your patient when their condition may affect their ability to drive

1. The history – you need to find out if this was self-harm or an attack. The police need not be informed for the former.

2. In the case of the latter, inform a senior colleague. Advise them you think the police should be informed in the interests of the safety of both patients and staff.

3. If you are responsible for informing the police, DO NOT disclose the patient's information at this stage, it is unnecessary. All the police need to be aware of is the incident.

The police arrive and wish to see the patient, but you feel the patient is not up to it. What next?

Your duty of care is to the patient and you should explain this to the police. When you feel the patient is ready, you can then ask them whether they wish to speak to the police.

A crime has been committed, but the patient is unconscious so you can't gain consent to reveal their details to the police. What should you do?

You can disclose confidential information as required by law and in the public's best interests. This is because others may be at risk of injury and/or it may aid prosecution for the crime (GMC 2009c). With any matters concerning confidentiality you should be seeking advice from the consultant in charge. Disclosing confidential information should never be rushed. Finally, if you are required to disclose anything, you must protect yourself by recording all the reasons for information disclosure in the patient's notes.

You find out that this is a domestic dispute and the victim does not want to press charges. What should you do?

Whilst it is appropriate to ask patients to disclose information necessary for their protection, you should abide by a competent adult's refusal if the risk of harm is only to themselves and not to others. However, you should warn them of the risks if they do not consent to disclose. You should also give them ways to seek help themselves, e.g. by informing them about domestic violence support groups. If children were involved in this case of domestic violence, however, you would be obliged to disclose the information to social services (GMC 2009d: Paras

51–56). Again, it is important to reiterate that, whilst you should be aware of what to do in difficult situations concerning confidentiality, you should always seek senior advice.

Confidentiality and the under eighteens

If a child is having an operation, it is best practice to have consent from both parents, but legally you only need one person with authority to give permission to treat. In an emergency, you don't need permission at all, as you can operate in the child's best interests. If there is a conflict that cannot be resolved informally, consult a senior as they may need to inform the legal department. Your trust will have a local policy on this, so it is advisable to familiarise yourself with it early on – or at least know where to access the information. Any decision made to act in a patient's best interests must be able to stand up if challenged.

Can a young person be seen without a parent?

Ideally a young person should have someone with them. However, you would never want to give them the impression that they could not get medical help – especially if it is something important that they do not feel comfortable telling their parents about (see Figure 2.3). You may also want to see them on their own if you suspect there is something odd about the family dynamics. Always offer a chaperone for any physical examination if they are on their own and record whether they accept or decline.

Note: divorce or separation does not make any one parent less responsible for their child.

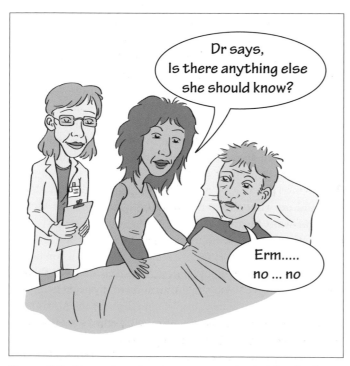

Figure 2.3 Recognise when teenagers may be holding back

What about a young person under sixteen years who wants contraception, an abortion or an STI check without their parents knowing?

This scenario is more likely to present working as a foundation doctor either on a GP or GUM rotation. It is recommended that you treat a young person in their best interests, provided that you cannot persuade them to talk to their parents and that they fully understand both the advice and the consequences. You may be recognising a pattern here, but always seek advice from a more experienced colleague; your job is to flag up situations like this to them so they can be handled in the most appropriate manner. This does not make your role any less important however as you do not recognise where issues can arise, then problems may occur. Your job as an FY1 includes gathering as much information as possible to pass onto your seniors.

How do you recognise potentially abusive or seriously harmful sexual activity in a young person?

This is an important distinction to make as often you will see teenagers under sixteen in relationships with an older partner (see Figure 2.4).

Examples of when you should consider sharing information are where (GMC 2011a: 28):
• The young person is too immature to understand.
• A big difference in age is ringing alarm bells!
• The partner is in a position of trust – e.g. the young person's teacher.
• There is a force/threat suggesting emotional, psychological or physical pressure.
• Drugs and/or alcohol are involved.
• The child is under 13 years (under 12 years in Scotland).

Generally speaking, a young person may feel more relaxed about confiding personal information to you, as someone who has been involved early in their treatment. Respect this and try to get as much information as possible, as it may be the only opportunity. If you suspect something untoward, it is often best to get the parents involved – with the young person's permission of course. Beyond this, you may have to notify social services. Remember to record your concerns and justify any decisions made by your senior about the disclosure. You also need to be honest with the patient about the information you are disclosing.

You have concerns about a parent's ability to cope with their child, what should you do?

This scenario is more likely to present itself in A&E. For any patient who comes in with a serious domestic injury, mental health issue or a history of drug or alcohol abuse, you must check whether they have any children. It may be that you need to put in a referral for social services as these children could well be at risk and have fallen completely under the radar.

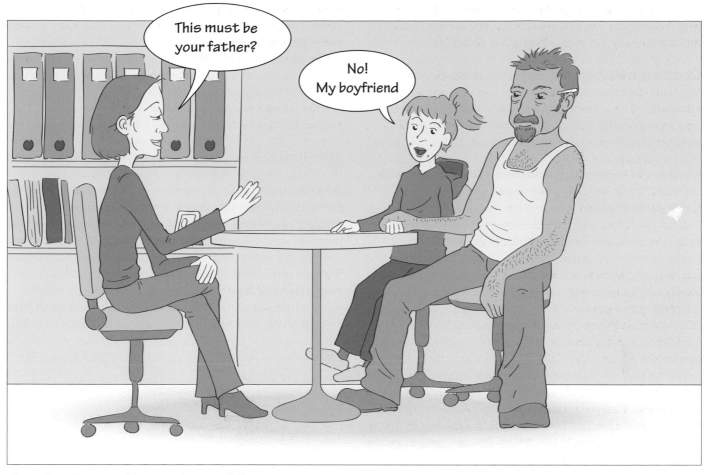

Figure 2.4 Be wary of inappropriate age differences

It is preferable that you gain consent from the parent when disclosing information to social services. Agree with the parent the information that you will share with social services. The information you will need is all on the proforma but will include:

- Patient details.
- Details of all the individuals in the household.
- What the problem is.
- Other agencies involved e.g. the school they go to, any health visitors.

It is not always necessary to get consent to contact social services. If you feel more harm would be caused to the child by not disclosing the information – for example if the parents would harm the child in some way – then you should not get consent and inform a senior straight away. In this instance, social services may be approached by telephone prior to sending the report in writing. This assessment is made on a case-by-case basis dependent upon the sense of urgency. Again, you would flag this up to a senior as this decision should be made by a more experienced colleague.

Jackie, ST1 *"A&E is the place you are safeguarding children . . . try to get as much information for social services as possible. It's a pain in the middle of the night on a busy shift, but it's important. You should also tell the parents about the referral. There is a box on the form asking whether you have told the parents. I wouldn't be happy submitting the form without the box ticked on my own judgement . . . . If I think getting consent is going to cause more harm than good, I get senior advice."*

For your reference, the GMC (2011b: para 60) advise the following order of preference for seeking advice:

1. An experienced colleague.
2. A named practitioner for child protection – your foundation clinical lead would help you with this.
3. A Caldicott guardian.
4. The GMC or another professional body (e.g. BMA, RCP) or defence body (non-EU).

Only the first two points are applicable to the FY1 as the foundation school would liaise with three and four on your behalf.

If social services call and ask for the medical records of carers of the child, what should you do?

You should consider any specific requests for information very carefully. Only very rarely would you disclose whole records and this would not be your decision to make. It is most appropriate to get your consultant to review any records, for which you would need the permission of the individual concerned. With any case, you should be aware that information can be disclosed if it is in the public interest. Although this is not your duty, it is important to be aware of it so that best practice is adhered to. If you see something wrong that could potentially breach confidentiality, you are expected to speak up: this is an aspect of 'integrity' that is often mentioned.

A young girl is diagnosed with cancer and her parents do not want you to tell her, what should you do?

Although breaking bad news is not the responsibility of an FY1, you should explore with the parents their reasons for not telling their daughter. You should explain to them that you should assess the capacity of the child and deliver information in a way they can understand. This is because children and young people usually want to know about their illnesses.

Exceptions to this are when:
- The information would cause "serious harm".
- The child specifically requests that someone else makes the decisions for them.

You should not withhold information unless the patient refuses knowledge of that information. The exception to this is if the information would cause "serious harm", which is more than making the patient upset or meaning that they might refuse treatment (GMC 2010). For example, if a child was particularly unwell, and the parents felt that giving the diagnosis would cause the child more harm and distress, you should get a senior to review the situation. However, you should also go and see the patient yourself and make your own judgement about the situation. If you agree that it would cause further harm, record this in the notes. The decision to withhold the information should be regularly reviewed and the information shared at the earliest possible opportunity. As a junior doctor, you should be aware of the patient's preferences at all times even though it will not be your sole responsibility to make these decisions. You are expected to advocate for your patients, and get as much information as possible to inform your colleagues.

Questioning professionalism

Samyami, FY2 *"Professionalism can quickly be lost . . . . I had a colleague in a bad mood who – rather than saying 'these bloods have been incorrectly labelled' – threw them at me, shouted on the ward in front of patients, relatives and everyone, before storming off. That's a massive question mark over their professionalism and it's moments like that where you completely lose credibility."*

If you realise that you have made a mistake and your integrity has been compromised, remind yourself that you are human and these things happen. There are however a few steps that you should take:

- Apologise to the person it affects: patient, colleague, relative.
- If it concerns a patient, document the apology in the notes and explain what problem was.
- The majority of mistakes that happen will be minor things; you can simply fill in a Clinically Adverse Event (CAE) form, learn from the mistake and move on.
- If the mistake is significant, inform your seniors.
- Complete a reflection piece within your eportfolio.

Tom, FY2 *"If you have made a mistake you always need to be honest with the patient. I made a mistake prescribing Warfarin. After I told my consultant, she said I needed to tell the patient. I went to tell the patient that we had accidently overcoagulated her and potentially put her at harm, but that we had corrected it and she was now within range. The patient hadn't come to any harm but I wanted to let her know . . . . She was fine with it. The next day her daughter came up to me, clearly very angry. She told me that she had lost all faith in doctors because of this incident. That was pretty hard to hear. I still think it was the right thing to tell the patient – not because the consultant told me to – but because it showed me that there was a consequence of my mistake, even though I hadn't harmed her."*

How should I learn from mistakes?

Charlotte, FY2 *"If you make a mistake you do need to reflect on it – and I know that's a cliché but you really have to. You have to be honest with yourself. Everyone makes mistakes; some are worse than others, but it's about how you deal with them. If you look into them seriously then you are unlikely to repeat them . . . . If you make a mistake once, you shouldn't really make the same mistake again."*

Expect to make mistakes; what's important is how you learn from them. Everyone groans at medical school at the mention of the word "reflection". Unfortunately, however, this is a crucial aspect of professionalism that is vital for your learning and personal development.

💡 **HERE ARE SOME TIPS FOR GOOD REFLECTION:**

- If something has happened that affected you – write it down!
- Self-regulation is an implicit aspect of reflection; evaluate what you could have done better. Most of the time it is only you who will question your decisions.
- If you find a gap in your knowledge, address it; no one else will do it for you.
- Know the personal state you were in and the circumstances under which the mistake happened. How can you flag these up in the future?
- Talk to your peers about it; chances are they will have been through a similar experience.
- Less is sometimes more. Don't reflect because you feel you have to, reflect at times where you know you will learn from it and it will make a difference. It's not about ticking a box.

Mithun, Consultant Psychiatrist *"As a doctor, you have to be proud of being a professional, and part of being a professional is being good at what you do – that is of the utmost importance. As a junior doctor, learn the importance of not taking short cuts . . . taking an extensive history . . . having an inquisitive mind. Be self-critical, want to better yourself and be the best there is. Ask yourself constantly: what can I do to improve my weaknesses?"*

TOP 5 TIPS ON PROFESSIONALISM:

1. Be conscious of your image as a professional within your personal life.

2. Stop and think before you share information.

3. If you are unsure at any point, consult a senior for advice.

4. If something goes wrong, find out what happened, then apologise to all those concerned.

5. Reflect on the important things that you know you can learn something from.

3 Pressures and prioritising

Carl, FY2 *"I really cannot stress the importance of organisation enough. You may think a lot of what you do goes unnoticed, but it is well appreciated. As soon as you have a house officer that is not organised it really becomes apparent . . . especially on surgical ward rounds . . . they have to run very quickly. If you are not on top of it they will notice."*

As far as coping with pressure is concerned, a foundation doctor is expected to:
- Work under pressure and remain calm and in control.
- Have effective coping mechanisms for stress.
- Demonstrate good judgement under pressure.
- Remain resilient and not give up easily.
- Deal with difficult situations and manage the unexpected.
- Know where to seek support.
- Deliver good time-management.

The common pressures which present themselves in foundation placements include:
- Probity
- Ward rounds
- Discharges
- Prescribing
- Consenting patients
- Learning and career development

Probity

Like integrity, probity is a word frequently bandied around the healthcare profession with assumed understanding. To be explicit, probity is about being honest and trustworthy and acting with integrity at all times, especially when under pressure. The following examples are experiences where probity has been challenged:

Mike, FY2 *"The patient's family did not want alcohol as the cause of death to be written on the death certificate. They became quite irate as they did not feel this was relevant. After speaking to the registrar – who confirmed it must be recorded – I went to explain to the family that I could not omit the information because that would be falsifying a document that I had a professional and legal obligation to fill out truthfully. They appreciated I took the time to find out all the information before discussing the death certificate with them and accepted my explanation."*

This is an example of external pressures being put on you by people asking you to falsify information. Another point on probity is being honest and trustworthy with respect to your colleagues:

Jeff, Consultant *"It was around Christmas time and one of the registrars asked to swap his New Year's Eve shift for Christmas Eve. Ordinarily this is quite a good switch. The registrar swapping had to rearrange a few family things but did it as a favour to his colleague. Two days before New Year's Eve the registrar who swapped rings and says 'you have to do New Year's Eve now because I have family coming that I forgot about'. This was rude and so unbelievably out of order. Ordinarily we wouldn't hear about such matters but this was so inappropriate, we were all appalled – suffice to say he would not be getting a reference from anyone in our department! Nobody trusted this person and it wasn't long before he moved on. After all there's nothing that should stop you from being on call, even if you had a holiday booked – we would expect you to get a later flight."*

SOME KEY THINGS TO REMEMBER ABOUT PROBITY WHEN UNDER PRESSURE:

- Document EVERYTHING: legally speaking if it's not written down, it didn't happen!
- Always read BEFORE you sign.
- Always be honest – that extends to being honest with your colleagues (see Figure 3.1).
- Remember that being trustworthy is integral to gaining respect.

Ward rounds

Sarah, FY1 *"There's always pressure, particularly on surgical ward rounds. They can be really rushed, but you have to remember that the consultant and specialist registrars have lots of other things to do. If you mess up the ward round in the morning, it messes up their whole day and can leave them in a really bad mood . . . . Being organised is really the key."*

Understand that as an FY1 you effectively run the team from the bottom up; you are the eyes on the floor. A large part of your role is clerical and, as the ward junior, you need to ensure the ward round runs smoothly. You will be expected to fill in the relevant gaps of each clinical case for the consultant as their commitments may mean they are unable to see the patient every day.

The Situational Judgement Test at a Glance, First Edition. Frances Varian and Lara Cartwright.

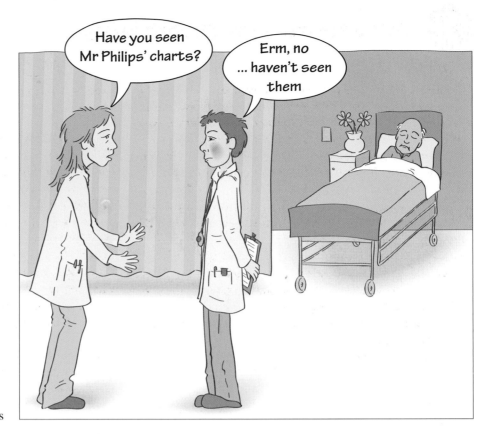

Figure 3.1 Be honest with your colleagues

💡 TIPS FOR A SUCCESSFUL WARD ROUND:

- Get to the ward at least 30 minutes before the round starts to prepare the notes.
- Know where your patients are.
- Ask the nurses whether there were any problems overnight.
- Have a system for writing the notes: date, time, ward, area and those present are the basic essentials.
- Summarise patient information before the round starts: the patient's observations now and when they came in, background, presenting complaint and results of any investigations.
- Know how to access bloods and images quickly.
- Remember to write your jobs in two places – in the notes and on your list – otherwise you might forget to do them.
- If you are unsure of the plan made, repeat it back to check. There is nothing more irritating for the consultant than having their management plan messed up, or you calling them later in the day to say "what did you actually mean by that?" Always clarify at the outset.

Patient discharge

There is huge pressure from the nurses and ward clerks to discharge patients. However, your priorities as a doctor are different from those of your colleagues who are expected to prioritise patient flow. Whilst you should support your colleagues and respect their roles, you must have an appropriate plan that completes the clinical journey such that patients are neither lost in the system, nor return to hospital (hopefully!).

> **Charlotte, FY2** *"Discharges can take a long time – often because you are multi-tasking (see Figure 3.2). Nurses will be asking you questions, physios asking you questions, OTs asking questions . . . your attention is constantly divided so what should take five minutes ends up taking thirty."*

Discharge letters may be dull but they are highly important. If they are not done properly, mistakes can lead to the patient getting lost in the system and not being followed-up, the GP not receiving the right information, the patient not getting the right medication . . . .The list goes on. Here's an example:

> **Priya, FY2** *"I had just joined a different hospital and I didn't know their policy on prescribing Warfarin on discharge was different. I prescribed it on the system, but didn't realise Warfarin had to be prescribed in the little yellow book for it to be dispensed. It wasn't until the nursing home rang me that I realised my mistake. I apologised and someone came to collect the prescription in the yellow book. From now on I always check the simple things when I move to a new hospital."*

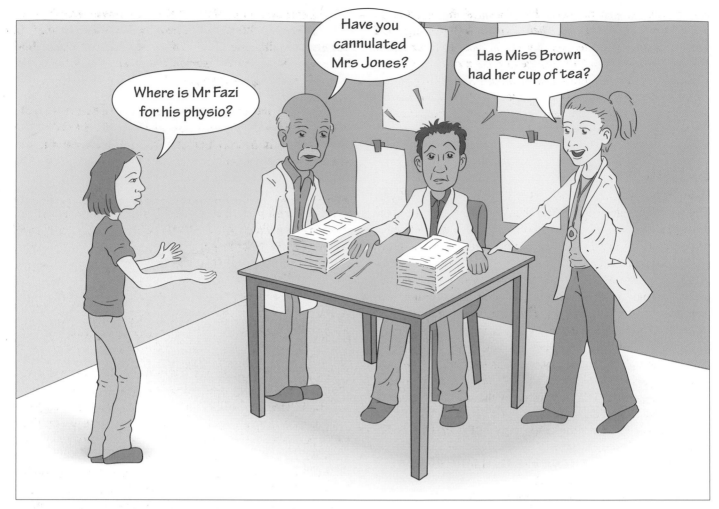

Figure 3.2 Try to avoid distractions when writing discharge summaries

What if a patient wants to self-discharge?

This would typically be against medical advice. In that case you should contact the patient's GP in person as the patient is at high risk of further illness. The GP can also set about trying to get in touch with the patient.

If the patient is a child, the situation is different. You can always stop them, or their parents, from trying to self-discharge provided you feel it is in the child's best interests to remain in hospital. You can do this by calling security in hospital, or the police if the patient is outside the hospital (in which case social services should also be notified).

🗣️ **Jackie, ST1** *"Although parents have the right to self-discharge; they don't have that same right concerning their child. One child was referred in from their GP with an exacerbation of asthma as his sats were 90%. I gave him an inhaler and his sats had improved, but I wanted to keep an eye on him as I wasn't completely happy for him to go home. His mum wasn't concerned and his sats were back up so she took that to mean he was fine. She said she had been waiting long* *enough and wanted to leave. I still wanted the registrar to review him though so I asked her to sign a self-discharge as I wasn't happy. I then pleaded that she at least wait for a new inhaler, but she left before even getting the medicine. If I was concerned about the child's asthma status I would have got the police to bring them back, but I wasn't overly concerned. I spoke to the registrar who suggested I contact the GP to get the medicine to them – which I did."*

Prescribing

Prescribing mistakes cost the NHS £500 million annually in England and Wales (DH, 2001). Nationwide, 5–7 % of acute medical admissions are due to prescribing errors, 50% of which are attributed to just four drugs: antiplatelets (16%), diuretics (16%), non-steroidal anti-inflammatories (11%) and anticoagulants (8%) (Howard et al. 2007). Prescribing should be considered as the most hazardous area for a junior doctor. Whilst you would never attempt a high-risk practical procedure without supervision, prescribing can be equally harmful – and you carry this out unsupervised from day one (Maxwell and Walley 2003). Strikingly, 90% of the prescribing done in any one hospital is by junior doctors; typically for paracetamol, morphine or metoclopramide (DH 2000). Learn the common mistakes now, so you don't make them.

The British Pharmacological Society (BPS 2010) lists ten principles of good prescribing:

1. Know WHY you are prescribing the drug. What is it for? How will it benefit your patient?

2. Know the patient's drug history (including OTC medications) and allergies.

3. Consider individual factors, e.g. age, pregnancy, kidney failure.

4. Elicit ideas, concerns and expectations (ICE)! Yes, that all important aspect of establishing a doctor–patient partnership is crucial for compliance.

5. Choose the best medicine for the patient considering: formulation, dose, frequency, route, duration and of course . . . cost.

6. Adhere to national, and local, guidance. Put into practice the textbook answer you use when your consultant asks you about antibiotic choice: *"I would use the one given in local hospital guidelines."*

7. Be aware of the common prescribing errors so you can avoid them e.g. write units, not U.

8. Monitor the medication and know how to report adverse drug reactions. Each BNF has a yellow card in the back which can be filled out and sent to the Medicine and Healthcare Products Regulatory Agency (MHRA). Alternatively you can access the MHRA online (MHRA 2012) and report side effects directly.

9. Document your reasons for prescribing and communicate these to patients, their carers and colleagues.

10. Only prescribe within your limitations, seek help early and get calculations double-checked.

Lorraine, ITU sister *"The two-person check is so important. We are all human and anyone can make a mistake . . . . You can listen without hearing and see without looking as well. The two-person check means you look at it, think about it and see it properly."*

Learn to be meticulous about prescribing and double-check. Names, doses and frequency should be legible. DO NOT DO ANYTHING BEYOND YOUR COMPETENCE even if you feel pressured to do so.

Never guess when prescribing; if you are unsure, ask a senior. Remember not to PANIC (see Figure 3.3) and you should avoid the common pitfalls:

- **Prescription** ⟶
- **Allergies**
- **Notes**
- **Interactions**
- **Clear**

- Right Drug
- Right Dose
- Right Route
- Right Patient

• PRESCRIPTIONS should always include the identity of the patient, the drug name, dose, frequency and start/finish dates. Eighty-five per cent of the errors that occur happen at the prescribing stage (Lesar et al. 1997) so check the British National Formulary (BNF) or ask someone for advice.

• Always ask about ALLERGIES and record any information on the chart properly. Do not write NKDA, use 'nil' or 'unknown'. Some consultants interpret NKDA as a sign that you simply haven't bothered to ask the question.

• Only in rare situations (i.e. an emergency) would you order a verbal prescription; hence, always write them up in the NOTES and on the drug chart beforehand to avoid mistakes.

• When prescribing multiple medications, be aware of INTERACTIONS and potential side effects. Furthermore, always take a full drug history. If the patient is unable to give you one, ask whether the ambulance brought anything in, or contact their GP.

• Finally, be CLEAR and write in CAPITALS when writing prescriptions, use the generic drug name –e.g. Ibuprofen instead of Nurofen – and write units correctly – i.e. microgram not mcg. Have a clear signature and remember the date, month and year. Be clear in communicating "your instructions to colleagues" rather than vice versa and, most importantly, be clear about your limitations. Always seek help early where patient safety is concerned.

Sally, FY1 *"I prescribed the wrong medication once. I was supposed to prescribe Metronidazole for bacterial vaginosis, but instead I prescribed Metformin!! The dosage,*

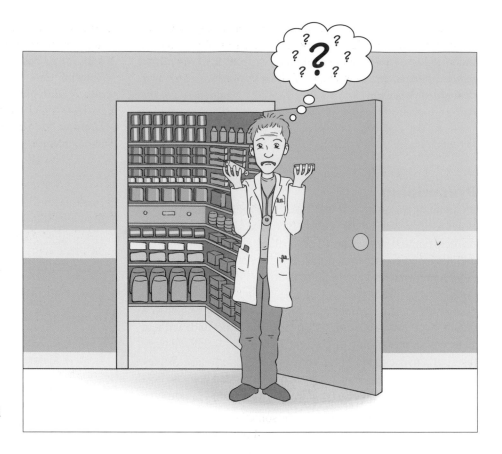

Figure 3.3 Try not to PANIC when faced with a difficult prescription

frequency and patient details were all correct, and I entered the correct drug name in the patient records, but I just wrote the wrong drug name on the prescription. Thankfully I had written "No Alcohol", and this alerted the pharmacist to the error so the patient received the correct medication in the end. Although this seems like one small error, its ramifications are huge. What if I had written Morphine instead of Metformin and the pharmacist had not realised? Then the patient would have been instructed to take 200mg of MST twice a day, with horrific consequences! It's likely the mistake occurred because I was chatting to the nurse as I wrote the prescription. Now I always take great care when prescribing, and double check what I've written."

If you make a mistake when prescribing, the Medical Protection Society (MPS, 2011) recommends the following actions for righting the wrong:
1. Explain what has happened to the patient and apologise.
2. Analyse the potential effects of the mistake and correct accordingly.
3. Apologise to any colleagues involved.
4. Fill in a CAE form so that lessons can be learned.

Paul, FY2 *"There was a lady on the medical ward who was diagnosed with a pulmonary embolus and was being Warfarinised. She had been given loading doses and was slow to get into range. Her INR hadn't been checked for 3 days and I had been asked to dose the Warfarin. It was 4.30 p.m. and I knew that if I took the bloods, I would have to hand it over for somebody else to dose. Her last INR was 1.3 and she'd had 3 doses since so I figured it would be OK. I dosed her and put a request out for the phlebotomist to take some bloods so that it would be ready for the next morning to accurately dose it. The INR came back as 10.7! We had to give her Vitamin K to reverse it. The patient didn't come to any harm and I explained to her what happened, but I am much more rigorous about prescribing Warfarin now and I don't take shortcuts."*

Consent

As consent is such a huge topic, this book breaks it into more manageable chunks. Capacity and not being able to consent are considered in Chapter 4. This section covers consent from the perspective of patients with capacity and the different pressures they may create.

For the most part, as a junior, the consent you gain will be implied or verbal. For example, gaining consent for venepuncture is easy; most of the time the patient will stick their arm out without you having to say anything. At other times, you would simply give a brief explanation of the ins and outs of the process. Tying together issues of confidentiality and implied consent, however, complicates the matter – particularly regarding the disclosure of information to relatives. The informal nature of a phone call or a family member approaching you at the ward desk can be challenging. Take stock of the situation first, and then make your judgement call.

Carl, FY2 *"As a house officer you are on the ward all the time and the patients and family will see you as their doctor because of that. The family will often come to you at the desk whilst doing discharges to ask how their family member is. If you know that they have a good relationship with your patient and have been involved in their care from the outset, then you can disclose some information. You have to be sure it's OK, though, as anyone could just walk in without even seeing the patient and ask how they are. You can't disclose in that instance, so don't feel pressured to do so. However, if disclosure includes important information such as diagnosis or sensitive investigations then you must always check if the patient is happy for you to disclose."*

What if I am asked to gain written consent for something I'm unsure of?

Being asked to gain written consent for a procedure that you are not so comfortable with may be something you are faced with as a junior. The way you manage this is important. The GMC (2008a) recommends that the responsibility for consent lies with the person doing the procedure. If someone delegates gaining consent to you, they are still responsible. Thus, whoever delegates the responsibility to you should make sure you are familiar with and understand the procedure and the benefits and risks involved. In this case you have two options:

1. Explain you don't yet have the experience but that you would like the opportunity to learn.
2. Begin the consent process and do what you can, leaving the formal signing to a more experienced colleague.

Judgement in this situation has to be made on the basis of your own knowledge, recognising where your limitations are. If you feel comfortable explaining some aspects of the procedure, then the second option is preferable. This assists the consent process but leaves the formalities to your more experienced colleague. In this situation you need to have a good relationship with your senior and to be sure that they will meticulously go over the information with the patient before signing the form. In reality, there are only a few surgical procedures for which you yourself will obtain consent and these will vary from locality to locality.

What should I do if a patient doesn't want to know?

Sharing information and knowing how much to share is central to good decision-making, but difficult to gauge. This can be daunting at first. The GMC (2008a) recommends tailoring all discussions to the patient without assuming the information they want. Ultimately you should:

1. Find out why they don't want the information.
2. Respect their decision not to have the information, BUT
3. Give them enough to gain consent: e.g. why you are doing it, a brief description of the procedure, any serious risks involved and whether they will have any pain afterwards.
4. If they won't have even the basic information, write down that this is what has happened and explain to them what that means. For example, this may mean that their consent is not valid.

What if a patient with capacity wants someone else to decide?

If the patient has capacity, the bottom line is that no one else can make the decision for them. The GMC (2008a) recommends that you:

1. Explain that it is important that they understand the options and the implications of any treatment.
2. Find out why they don't want the information.
3. Iterate that their consent won't be valid if they do not have this information.

What about consent in an emergency?

The GMC (2008a) recommends that you should gain oral consent in these circumstances but the patient should still have all the information they need. Record this in their notes. If the patient is unable to consent then you can act in their best interests (see Chapter 4).

Ultimately you should recognise that, as a junior, you have only been qualified for a short time. Issues of consent are highly complex and the consequences of one decision over another are largely beyond what you can see. You must share this responsibility and find someone with more experience to give you advice. If something such as a breach of confidentiality happens because you have not gained consent, it cannot be taken back. Nevertheless, the right actions can be sought afterwards.

Amit, FY2 *"I was looking after an elderly gentleman with hypercalcaemia who was intermittently confused. His daughter was heavily involved in his care. She asked one of the nursing staff about his CT results. And the nurse – without checking with anyone – said 'Yes, we're doing some further investigations to confirm whether the mass is cancer'. I looked up and thought what have you done?! We hadn't told the patient yet because he was intermittently confused, but between episodes he seemed to have capacity. We then had the situation where the relative had been told and the patient didn't know. The daughter then spoke to me and asked me to keep it from him because she thought he wouldn't take it very well and he had been quite down recently. To be asked by a relative not to tell the patient is completely wrong. I spoke to my consultant and we had a team meeting with the nursing staff to discuss the breach . . . in the end the patient was OK with it."*

Learning and career development

🗣 **Samyami, FY2** *"Never forget you are there to learn – not just to complete jobs and discharge patients – that way, you'll really enjoy your foundation training."*

Training whilst doing a job means that pressures in terms of learning and career development are constant. With some tips and good time-management however this can be something to enjoy.

A foundation doctor is expected to:
- Have a desire and enthusiasm for continued learning.
- Take responsibility for their own development.
- Learn from others and from others' experiences.
- Be open and accepting of feedback – appraisals are a key time for this.
- Have a desire and willingness to teach others – medical students are usually there for you to impart your wisdom to them.

There are plenty of opportunities for learning beyond your protected teaching time. These can be considered within three broad areas:
- Informal
- Procedural
- Teaching

🗣 **Mohammed, Consultant Surgeon** *"Know what you want from your career so you can target the areas of interest and make the most of experiences you know you won't have again in the future . . . . I made the most of medicine because I knew I wasn't going to do it again."*

Informal opportunities

Remember to learn on the job (see Figure 3.4).
- Go down to theatre and practice your suturing; the surgeons will be more than happy to have you.
- Engage in meetings by presenting cases or clinically adverse events.
- Get involved with an audit, and do it early! You will have to complete them throughout your career. The trick is to pick something simple; this will lessen the time pressure and make it easier to repeat.
- When you start a job, let your consultant and/or educational supervisor know what you want from the rotation and – if you know – from your career. This way they can offer you extra experience or direct you towards another team who can help.

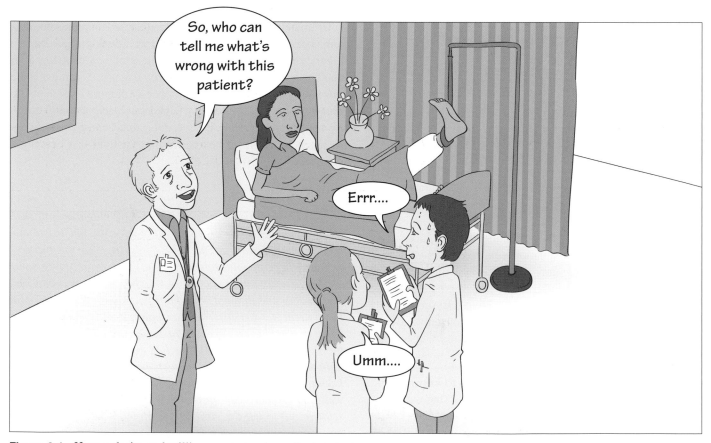

Figure 3.4 Have a desire and willingness to teach medical students

John, FY2 *"Ward teaching happens all the time. I pick up something new every day: new drugs and new indications, or changes to guidelines. I find that I learn things that I would never get from a book or even remember in a lecture – but the fact that I was told about it and then asked to prescribe it makes me remember it."*

Alice, FY2 *"Know that these two years are probably going to be the best two training years as you get to do a bit of everything. You should go into each of your rotations with an open mind and not think 'well I'm going to do surgery so I don't care about elderly medicine'. Every speciality you do is going to be important in terms of what you go on to do. If you pick up lots of little skills then you won't feel daunted about doing a different specialty; in that respect you should already have developed the practical skills to do the job."*

Procedural

Take every opportunity to learn new skills.
- Get as much practical experience as you can: go and see lumbar punctures, chest drains etc.
- If you have a quiet job and a lull in the day, remember that you are a trainee, so try to develop your skills in that time. Don't just chill out and have a coffee as you may not get another chance.

Carl, FY2 *"Your Registrar or SHO will always want to teach you, as they don't want to be the only person that can do something. Most jobs come with one or two specialist procedures that you should take the opportunity to learn. Once out of that job, you may never get that opportunity to gain that skill. I did a gastro job and I did 30 ascitic drains in four months. I feel confident now that I can do them on my own. If you can get one or two good transferable skills from every job, then you*

have done well in terms of learning opportunities – any more than that is perhaps unrealistic."

Teaching medical students

Nick, FY2 *"FY1s and FY2s give some of the best teaching as they still remember what it's like to be a medical student. Having been through finals, they know the level that you need to know. As a medical student you can overestimate what you really need to know and much of it you will never be asked in finals. Formally teaching students also forces you to brush up on knowledge that you haven't looked at over the past few months – though you would never admit this – so you learn as well!"*

Prioritisation

Fraz, FY2 *"If you are organised it allows you to be more efficient and prioritise more effectively. Prioritisation isn't easy at first, but it comes easier if everything else is organised in a timely fashion."*

For effective organisation and planning, as a foundation doctor you should:
- Manage and plan workload effectively.
- Display efficient time-management.
- Deliver tasks on time.
- Prioritise effectively and reprioritise where appropriate.
- Assimilate a range of information and identify key issues.
- Think creatively to solve problems.
- Be proactive and take initiative.
- Attend to detail.

Learning to prioritise your workload can be the hardest part of adapting to your foundation job. One particularly useful time-management tool – the Important/Urgent Grid – is described by Covey (2004) see Figure 3.5.

	Urgent	Non-urgent
Important	**'Critical activities'** • Sick patient • Answering your bleep • Meeting deadlines e.g. appraisal, eportfolio	**'Important goals'** • Patient safety • Helping out colleagues • Discharge • Death certificates • Clinical audits • Taking a break
Not important	**'Interruptions'** • Answering the ward telephone • Responding to colleagues interrupting you	**'Distractions'** • Checking email • Social networking • Jobs you could delegate to others e.g. bloods, drawing up drugs

Figure 3.5 Important/urgent grid (adapted from Covey 2004)

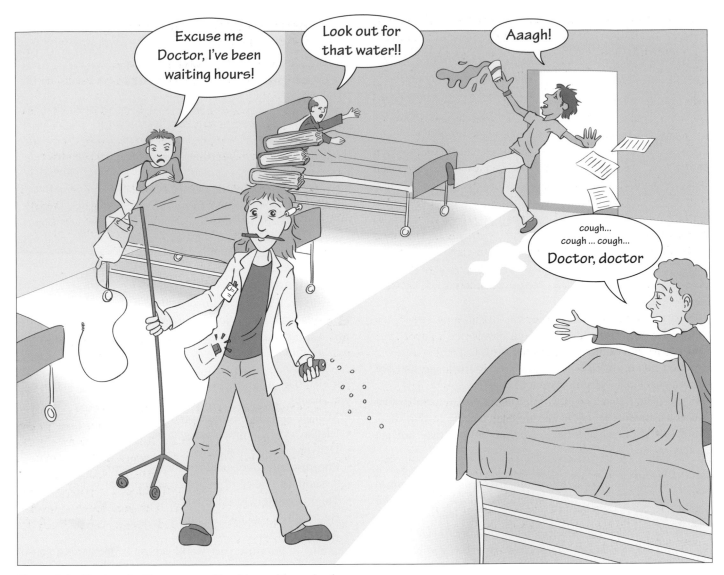

Figure 3.6 Try to prioritise your workload to avoid overload

Covey (2004) describes a grid formation of tasks divided with respect to urgency and importance. This system allows you to prioritise tasks more efficiently and use your time more effectively, leading to a more successful and less stressful working day. It's easy to prioritise tasks that are both urgent and important (top left quadrant). These "critical activities" include the "quick wins" and general buzz of "getting the job done". However, this can lead to a feeling of being constantly busy, but unproductive overall (Figure 3.6).

Covey (2004) highlights how you must focus on the important and non-urgent tasks as well as the urgent. Prioritisation will therefore be more successful if you concentrate your time in the "important goals" area of the grid (top right quadrant). A few examples of these tasks are included in Figure 3.5 but the list is by no means definitive. While on your clinical placements, consider arranging tasks in this format to aid your prioritisation; starting early means you can hit the ground running when you qualify.

Sarah, FY1 *"After a ward round I sit down with all the notes and the list of jobs and put them in order of priority of urgency: urgent, important and those that can wait. Radiology requests are usually the first thing I do, then discharges, as I know nurses are under pressure to discharge patients."*

If at any stage you feel "critical" tasks are overloaded, consider the reasons why. Some will be "crisis" items which could not have been foreseen; however, some might have been prevented from becoming urgent if they had been tackled at an earlier stage. For example, if your appraisal is imminent and you haven't completed your self-reflection, ask yourself if you could not, realistically, have done this earlier to avoid the additional stress? Generally speaking, if you spend a high percentage of your working day tackling tasks in this quadrant, stress levels will be high. At this point you should consider asking for help, as you will either need to find another way to manage your workload or to raise the issue that the workload is simply too much for one person to handle.

"Distractions" should be considered as time-stealers which prevent you from achieving your goals. Question whether such tasks can be delegated, rescheduled or simply avoided: should you really be checking your email for the tenth time that morning? These could also be things that others want you to do for them, rather than things which contribute to your own goals. Saying no politely but firmly at an early stage is one strategy, but you must also remember that teamwork is about give and take. See Chapter 6 for considering other team members' roles.

Finally, interruptions are difficult to avoid, especially when working on the wards. If you find that this is causing particular delay, consider whether you need to find a different place to do your paperwork, or to redirect some of it elsewhere. Part of being a good team-player, however, is being open to interruptions. In this respect, the most important thing to remember is to make sure your priorities are flexible:

Fraz, FY1 *"If you're working on call on a surgical rotation and you're the only FY1 available, you have to quickly prioritise. For example, if you have cannulas and a patient crashing; just because the cannula is number one on your list doesn't mean you do it, you have to switch around and swap your priorities."*

With respect to prioritising patients, every patient should be assessed in terms of their CLINICAL needs as this determines their investigations and treatment. On a side note, the GMC (2009a) stresses how these priorities should never be affected by your personal views of the patient; hence even if they are a repeat attender or behaving badly, you prioritise their clinical needs regardless. See Chapter 5 for additional information on patients.

As a medical student, you are well schooled in recognising the sick patient; it is the more day-to-day tasks that can be initially hard to prioritise.

Nick, FY1 *"Prioritisation is key: for patient safety more than anything. It's hard initially as you're unsure which jobs to do first and how fast to do them. I remember my first week as an FY1, I clerked a patient in with hemiplegia and I had bloods, an ABG . . . a whole list of jobs were just piling up with no idea where to start. I sought advice from the FY2 and she knew straight away which ones to put at the top of the pile."*

Bleeps

At any one time on the wards you could potentially have two bleeps:
- Your personal bleep
- An on-call bleep
- This should NOT be SOMEONE ELSE'S bleep!

On-call bleeps are notoriously difficult to prioritise – especially in medicine where, in smaller localities, you may be the only doctor covering all the medical wards in the hospital. At the same time as prioritising your patients, you also have to find time to attend to your own bodily functions: peeing, eating, etc. Ideally, you should not hand over your bleep to another colleague as this is effectively handing over responsibility for your patients to them.

Sarah, FY1 *"On call in medicine you get bleeped continuously. My colleague handed his bleep to a nurse whilst he had a very quick pee on call last Saturday and during this short time his bleep went off 13 times! The nurses bleeping you will want to get whatever they are asking for done immediately, and often will be quite insistent that you need to do this cannula NOW, despite the fact you are currently singlehandedly juggling a septic patient, a pulmonary embolism and an acute exacerbation of asthma – as I was 2 weeks ago. In this situation you will be stressed, hungry and tired. Trying to be firm about the priority of a cannula but simultaneously remaining polite is really, really hard. And it is a daily example for junior doctors on the importance of professionalism."*

There are a few situations in which it is acceptable to handover or 'silence' your bleep, these include:
- During handover (see Chapter 6).
- When breaking bad news (see Chapter 4).
- During protected teaching time.

An important point to note about breaking bad news is that patients can see you ignoring your bleep if it goes off

– demonstrating that you are giving them your undivided attention. Hence, not silencing your bleep can be a positive thing and should be judged specific to the situation. Your personal bleep should be with you at all times and answered in a timely manner. The exception to this is during protected teaching time. Here you are usually asked to hand in your bleep before entering the lecture theatre to ensure your learning is uninterrupted. Ignoring a bleep without very good reason is not acceptable, as this could seriously compromise patient care.

TOP 5 TIPS ON PRESSURES AND PRIORITISING:

1. Be honest, clear and up to date with all information.
2. Take responsibility for – and pride in – your job role.
3. Be systematic with your jobs list and prioritise according to urgency and importance.
4. Adapt quickly to situations.
5. Remember you are learning: so seek every opportunity to do so.

4 Effective communication

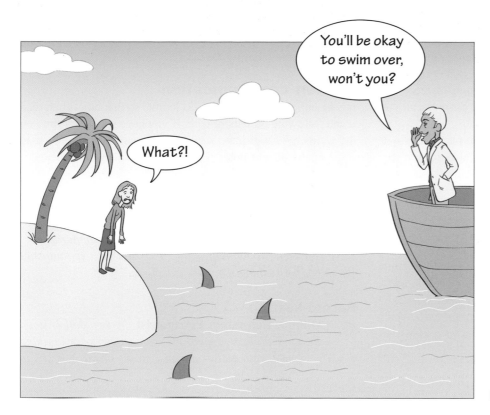

Figure 4.1 Don't belittle patients' concerns

Mary, patient *"A good doctor is able to communicate well: be comprehensible, direct, and sensitive to my responses and my needs as the patient. Having patience is also key . . . for example, when presented with oedema around the ankles, saying 'it's not exactly life-threatening is it?' isn't particularly helpful!"* (see Figure 4.1)

With respect to effective communication, a foundation doctor is expected to:
• Communicate with patients, relatives and colleagues effectively and sensitively.
• Adapt their style of communication to individual needs and context.
• Ensure they have all the relevant information before communicating.
• Ensure the surroundings are appropriate when communicating.
• Seek clarification to gain and check understanding.
• Readily answer questions and keep patients, relatives and colleagues updated.

Five principles for good communication
The British Medical Association (BMA 2004a) recognises that a doctor must have competent written and oral communication skills. But what constitutes "good" communication skills? Kurtz (1989) outlines five principles for success:

1. Interaction rather than dictation: in other words, a two-way conversation.

2. Reduce uncertainty by allowing the patient to ask questions.

3. Plan and think about the outcomes. Know beforehand what you want to achieve from the conversation or what you want to convey to others in writing.

4. Dynamic: be flexible from one patient to another and be responsive to individual needs. You will encounter a wide variety of patients for which you must adapt your approach.

5. Helical: what one person says influences another and so on and so forth, so that the conversation evolves. This can be challenging, as it requires you to adapt your thoughts to the patient's response. Whilst you may enter the conversation having a set number of points to cover, you may leave having taken a very different tangent.

The BMA (2004a) also list barriers to communication which are summarised below in order to help you evaluate your own communication skills. Do you find yourself falling into any of these traps?

• **Lack of understanding** of conversational interaction: see Kurtz's principles above.

• **Inadequate recognition** of non-verbal skills, including body language and the setting.

The Situational Judgement Test at a Glance, First Edition. Frances Varian and Lara Cartwright.

- Regarding communication as a **low priority**. Often all patients need is to feel listened to, and they will feel well cared for.
- **Not having the confidence** to communicate effectively.
- **Lack of clinical knowledge** about a condition. If you find yourself in this position, be honest with the patient and say that you don't know. It is not appropriate to deliver inaccurate information.
- **Human factors**: know yourself well enough to recognise fatigue and stress. Act on this accordingly: for example, all you may need is a 10-minute break.
- **Personality differences**: understanding your personality will help you communicate better. Moreover, you also need to recognise the personality of others, i.e. patients, colleagues and relatives, to better communicate with them.

> **Sophie, FY1** *"Lack of communication can be a big issue – there are different types of doctors and different bedside manners (See Figure 4.2). Sometimes there can be paternalistic styles which are out of keeping with patient expectations and medical practice, and sometimes compassion is not shown. This can leave the patient quite upset. It's not that they are bad doctors, they just haven't communicated in the right way for that individual patient."*

The common complaints involving communication arise from three areas (BMA 2004a): patients not being involved in changes to their care; patients given conflicting information by different people (especially doctors and nurses); and clinical notes not being clear or not referred to appropriately. Good communication with colleagues and accurate record-keeping can resolve the latter two areas.

Written communication

It is essential that your writing is legible so that others can read it and follow up on patient care. If you have spent any time on the wards, you will have seen how difficult it can be to read some of the patient notes. Please think about your colleagues and try to write as clear as possible.

> **Rajen, ST4** *"We do audit notes for legibility. All entries should be signed including the GMC number. We will have words with doctors who fail to meet such standards . . . . Have you seen the nursing notes? They are always fantastic! We should be keeping the same standards."*

Record-keeping

> **Mithun, Consultant Psychiatrist** *"A key skill is good documentation. I expect everyone to write everything down – almost verbatim – not just to sit down and try to*

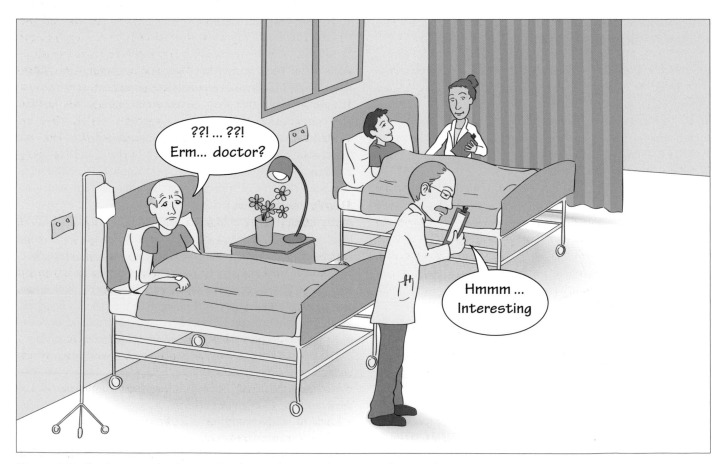

Figure 4.2 Good communication requires interaction . . . often all a patient needs is to be listened to

summarise things from perception. Verbatim is more powerful in psychiatry and carries more weight than summarising findings. Writing should be legible, and each entry dated with the patient's name and date of birth on every page. If it's not, and the continuation sheet is lost, you don't know where it's come from."

Good writing in the notes is part of communication. For the majority of the time, the purpose of writing is so that somebody else can read a summary of the patient's problems. If your writing is illegible, this may result in a patient's plan not being actioned.

💡 **TIPS FOR SUCCESSFUL DOCUMENTATION:**

(See Chapter 3 for tips on ward rounds and discharges):
• Always write in BLACK ink in the margin: date, time, ward and area.
• Always sign your name, print it and put your bleep and/or GMC number.
• Use only accepted, well-known and unambiguous abbreviations e.g. BP, HR, MEWS.
• Be thorough: Write LEFT not L. and RIGHT not R. – this is critical in surgery, taking off the wrong limb or removing the wrong organ is a 'should never happen' event.
• Be contemporaneous and NEVER retrospectively change notes.

🗣 **Tony, Consultant Surgeon** *"A peer of mine who worked in a dysfunctional department told me this story. A patient came in over the weekend and was seen by the locum registrar. The patient was a young lady with pyelonephritis who sadly died on the Monday. This registrar then went and wrote in the notes over the weekend AFTER the event . . . . He never worked in that hospital again."*

What else should you document?

🗣 **Sam, FY2** *"My first few months I forgot to document things half the time. Anything beyond routine jobs you should really document so try to get into this habit early. All discussions with relatives and other professionals . . . even informal discussions with OTs and physios. Put it down even if it seems obvious, especially if you are not around the next day to impart that information, as it may not be obvious to the ward cover or on-call doctor."*

There is a multitude of certificate and form-filling as an FY1. Routine elements considered here are: blood forms, clinical coding, death certificates and cremation forms.

Blood forms

🗣 **Sarah, FY1** *"Taking bloods is a great opportunity to sit down and have a chat with the patient; you get to develop your relationship with them and that means they get better quicker."*

🗣 **Carl, FY2** *"I always fill in everything on the blood form. There's nothing worse than having to re-bleed a patient . . . especially if they're difficult."*

💡 **THE FOLLOWING TIPS APPLY TO BLOOD REQUESTS:**

• All requests should be clinically indicated. Don't just tick boxes because you can.
• Think: is the information you have put on your form enough for the laboratory staff to be able to call you about an abnormal result? Blood tests mean little without the clinical context (Patel and Morrissey 2011).
• Fill in ALL the required information on the blood bottle and the form, otherwise it won't get processed and patient care will be compromised.
• Follow up the results: your test, your responsibility.

Clinical coding

This is something you may have heard described at medical school. You should have a good induction on coding at your trust when you start working, but here are some basics. Throughout the UK, the system is called the Kohner Medical Record (KMR). Coding involves putting every patient admitted – their diagnosis, co-morbidities and any procedures/treatments – into the computer (or on a written form in the front of their notes). This is an important form of communication because, if you miss something vital in the diagnosis (e.g. hypertension), then it may be missed at handover and so on throughout their care. The KMR is also important for population statistics and the allocation of resources, as the more patients the hospital treats with co-morbidities, the bigger the budget they are assigned. Finally, you should consider utilising this data as a valid selection method for a clinical audit (Patel and Morrissey 2011).

Death certificates

🗣 **Ahmed, FY1** *"I made a mistake certifying early on. It was for one of my patients who came in with a fall and died two weeks later from something unrelated. I didn't realise that, because she'd had a fall, she had to go to the coroner. The process was delayed as a result, so it's worth getting it checked."*

• Examine the patient thoroughly to confirm death. It has – very rarely – happened that a patient has woken up in the morgue!
• Remember to check for a pacemaker: this is important if they are being cremated.
• Understand there may be specific religious wishes that you need to be sensitive towards.
• To sign the death certificate you must have seen the patient alive at least 14 days prior to their death (ONS 2010).

- Know the circumstances in which a death needs to be discussed with the coroner (procurator fiscal in Scotland). Their duty is to decide whether to issue the certificate, order a post-mortem or start an inquest into the cause of death (Patel and Morrissey 2011).
- Be accurate about the cause of death. Ask advice from someone more senior as, if not done accurately, this can delay the whole process and the family cannot grieve in a timely manner.

Cremation forms

This is a paid professional duty and should be done in a timely manner to avoid delay for the family. Two people independently certify for cremation. The first person fills in part one and the second person – with 5 years' experience – fills in the second part. These forms need to match the death certificate, and it makes things smoother if you contact the person who signs part two to let them know that you have completed your section (Patel and Morrissey 2011). You should have identified the deceased; you should have seen them recently, and after death to confirm they do not have a pacemaker or radioactive device which could cause an explosion! Finally, you need to speak to the named nurse who was caring for the patient and was with them when they died as this information is required on the form.

Common errors in completing this form, which result in a delay for cremation and funeral for the family are (Ministry of Justice 2012):
- Not completing the questions in full.
- Missing out questions.
- Filling the form in incorrectly.
- Illegible handwriting.
- Discrepancies between the two parts on date and time of death.

Your local trust will have policy documents for you to view on death certificates and cremation forms which you should familiarise yourself with. If you want to look at the forms in the meantime, you can search for the Ministry of Justice website online or follow this link: http://www.justice.gov.uk/coroners-burial-cremation/cremation.

Verbal communication

Whilst oral communication skills require practice and self-reflection, there are some key points to consider regarding situations where communication can be difficult:
- Working with interpreters.
- Communicating with patients with a disability.
- Communicating your personal views.
- Communicating with difficult relatives.
- Breaking bad news.

Working with interpreters

Carl, FY2 *"It is difficult to refuse an offer from the family to translate, but if you feel uncomfortable about it, then you have to. I was working in a haematology clinic and had to disclose diagnoses such as lymphoma. With this, it was hospital policy to routinely test for HIV and Hepatitis B/C. Disclosing that information via a translator is hard enough, but if you are using a family member, then there is too great a potential for conflict. Because there is an emotional tie, there are a lot of potential for problems, and you can cause a lot of damage if you don't disclose in the right way. Also, if you are disclosing things like that in clinic, it is always better to have a chaperone."*

When you encounter a language barrier, try to arrange an interpreter. It is rarely appropriate to use a family member – except perhaps in an emergency where they can give you a history and medications. The problems with using a friend or relative are (Phelan 1995):
- Their views produce inaccuracies.
- They try to protect patients from bad news.
- They don't reveal side effects as they think compliance will be better.
- The patient may not want to disclose 'embarrassing' information to them.

Tony, Consultant Surgeon *"I remember a case 5 years ago of a chap who spoke Urdu and his daughter was translating for him. It was really important that he understood that he had a staghorn calculus in his left kidney that would eventually stop it working, as I wanted to take out his right kidney with the tumour in it. He wasn't that keen on treatment and said 'No I'll leave it'. The medical student then said – once they'd gone out: 'she just said "you've got a stone on the left and stone on the right, you need surgery" and didn't tell him what the matter was.' He therefore left with no idea of the importance of getting treatment so couldn't make an informed decision. It just shows how families can find it difficult to be objective and relay your issues straight across."*

The best options for interpretation are professional services such as the in-hospital translation service or telephone translation service. You should check what services are available at each trust.

> **SOME KEY TIPS FOR WORKING WITH INTERPRETERS:**
>
> (As suggested by Phelan [1995]):
> - Debrief the interpreter before and after the consultation.
> - Direct questions to the patient and maintain eye contact with them and not the interpreter.
> - Speak simply and pause to allow for translation.
> - Respond to non-verbal cues.
> - Check the patient's understanding.
> - Try to use the same interpreter for future interviews where possible.

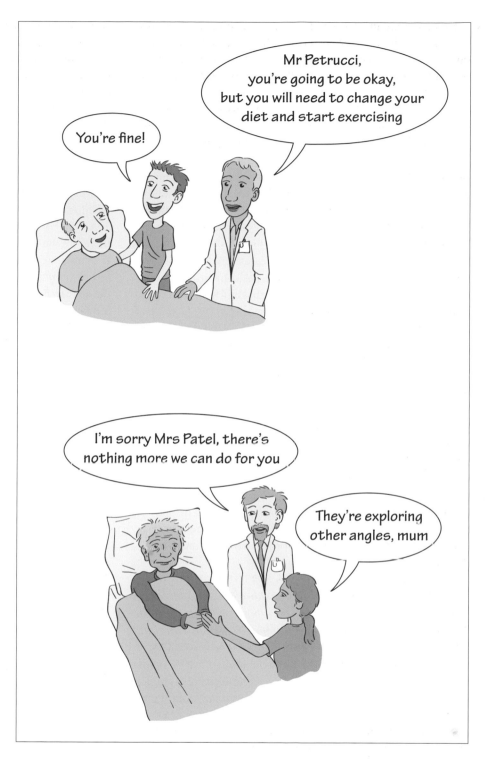

Figure 4.3 You should seek a professional interpreter where possible to avoid miscommunication

Another situation in which you may consider using an interpreter is when patients have a communication disability. Communication support includes: lip readers, British Sign Language (BSL) interpreters, deafblind interpreters, note takers, etc.. If communication support is needed, notice should ideally be given up to six weeks in advance (Directgov 2011).

Working with disability

Depending on the focus of the teaching, the distinction between impairment and disability may have already been drummed into you at medical school: so one more time is probably not going to hurt! Impairment is considered the actual physical or mental 'effect'. For example, someone who is obese may be unable to walk for more than fifty metres without resting, resulting in mobility restrictions. This impairment would extend to a disability if the effects meant the individual was unable to work or carry out their daily functions as usual for at least 12 months (ODI 2010). Disability is therefore determined by the effect of the impairment; defined by the Disability Discrimination Act (1995) as "a physical or mental impairment which has a substantial and long-term adverse effect on a person's ability to carry out normal day-to-day activities". This is why you must ask every patient how their condition (i.e. impairment) affects their day-to-day life. The social implications of an illness significantly affects your management of it. Without knowing about them, you cannot truly empathise with your patients.

Mental impairment can pose the greatest challenge to communication. The EHRC (2010) outline has some useful tips for communicating with patients with a disability to help avoid non-attendance and missed appointments:

1. Avoid "diagnostic-overshadowing" and seeing patients only in terms of their impairment. For example, a patient with autism may be behaving inappropriately because they are in pain rather than as a result of their impairment.
BUT ALSO
2. Recognise that impairment can lead to health inequalities that require special attention.

A patient with a learning difficulty should have the same access to healthcare services as everyone else. However, they should also receive full annual physical health assessments as research suggests they have a shorter life expectancy due to the higher risk of health inequalities. More time should be allowed for these assessments (and thorough physical examination) as impaired communication can impede history-taking (EHRC, 2010).

Nick, FY1 *"I had difficulties with a 35-year-old patient who – since birth – had no verbal communication. He was self-mobile and could care for himself, and his carer said he had an excellent quality of life (QOL) and was quite active. He came in with a severe pneumonia and, after maximum medical therapy, was still unwell. We called for an ITU opinion and they came down. After a short assessment they said 'no we won't take him'; deciding he had a poor QOL due to severe learning difficulties. I had to arrange for an Independent Mental Capacity Advocate (IMCA) to assess the situation. They laid out all the facts in order to make a decision and were brilliant. The patient recovered in the meantime thankfully."*

Some key learning points from this example are (EHRC 2010):
• Never make assumptions about a patient's experience of their disability. For example, not every deafblind patient will have a learning disability. Also, you should avoid attributing physical complaints to a psychological cause in a patient with known mental health problems.

• Never make assumptions about the personal life of a patient with a disability – they have the same potential for a sex life as everyone else.
• Find out and remember their preferred means of communication, e.g. writing everything down if they are deaf.
• Note any access requirements for future appointments: e.g., on discharge, are they able to find their way to their follow-up appointment in two weeks?
• Note any mobility requirements and make sure the nurses and healthcare assistants are also aware of them.
• Every effort should be made to understand patients' wishes whether or not they have capacity.

As an FY1, you will have first contact with patients and therefore the time to find out from them their individual needs. If communication is difficult, simply ask them how they wish to be communicated with and make sure this is relayed to all the staff so that the patient does not have to keep repeating their requirements. Some patients may have a "passport" for healthcare which has all the relevant information on their condition – take note of this.

Michael, GP *"Not speaking slowly and shouting are two key things you should never do! It's about understanding how the disability affects them. . . . As doctors, we are too often scared to talk about a disability but most people living with a disability are more than happy to talk about what that means."*

What about those patients who are newly diagnosed with a disability?

This is very important as patients get stigmatised and marginalised when labelled with a disability. The more you can support patients on wider social issues, the greater benefit you will be. Also note that time of diagnosis is crucial for every patient and must be handled with empathy, sensitivity and practicality to avoid any potential complaints.

As a doctor you will likely be asked about (EHRC 2010):
• Fit notes – you will probably be expected to write these for patients for discharge, and it is necessary to know how much time the patient will need for recuperation at home.
• Benefits and statements for home adaptations.
• Disabled parking badges.

If you are unsure, inform the patient about the EHRC (Equality Human Rights Commission). They give telephone advice and guidance on many issues ranging from reasonable adjustments employers are expected to make, to expectant parents and social housing providers. There are also other sites you can go to, such as Directgov, which has a wealth of information as well as applications for disability grants and blue badges (Directgov 2012). Knowing where to direct patients is equally as helpful as having all the answers yourself. In the interim, you can also ask for senior input, advice from the nursing staff or, if activities of daily living are concerned, advice from an occupational therapist.

Communicating personal views

- **Speak out if you see bad practice.**

  Colette, Consultant Surgeon *"Safety is very important. You must raise concerns as soon as possible . . . The consultant will not get annoyed about asking questions. They may get annoyed if you do not ask and something goes wrong."*

- **Be careful about the language you use – is it suitable for your audience?**

  Bill, Patient *"I had polymyalgia rheumatica and was on steroids for it. At the time I was seeing a young GP at the practice who I generally got on well with, but my ESR and CRP had been fluctuating. He admitted he had been 'bollocked' by the consultant rheumatologist at the hospital . . . . 'Bollocked' was his comment! As if I would ever use such a word . . . "*

- **Don't forget, no matter how well you know the patient, you are still their doctor.**

  Tony, Consultant Surgeon *"I once referred to the hospital as 'a hotel whilst recuperating' as you're without any need for intervention. That was taken as grossly offensive by the patient. This was a misjudgement of my rapport with the patient. I don't think I've got it as wrong as that since. The patient was very angry so I apologised and took a step back. I had been slightly too familiar... it had been a less formal doctor–patient conversation, but my description of using the hospital as a hotel didn't work for him and he took it as offensive rather than descriptive."*

- **Know your limitations, when to seek help, and when to have confidence in your skill set.**

  Carl, FY2 *"You need to decide how far you can manage something before you escalate it up . . . . That's the skill . . . working out the point at which you decide you are out of your depth, but not letting it get to that point before you make that decision. There is a fine balance between not shooting it straight up to the registrar without doing anything for that patient, and leaving it too late before you ask. You need to cut a balance to stabilise the patient and do all the necessary investigations. If you speak to the registrar and they say they don't need something, you can simply cancel the request. But if you ring them and say 'the patient is septic', and they ask what you have done and you haven't done even the initial investigations, they won't be very happy with you. That's your bread and butter really – doing the initial work-up. When you reach the point where you don't know where to go . . . then you should escalate it up."*

Communicating with relatives

Alice, FY2 *"Patients will have no idea where you are in the cycle of being a doctor. They won't be interested if it's your first day or tenth year as a doctor, they still expect a certain standard of you. Talking to patients and their relatives is one of the biggest challenges."*

In difficult, evocative and emotional situations you have to be really careful about the language you use and the clarity with which you provide explanations.

Samyami, FY2 *"I understand that this is your mum and you are very concerned and you have every right to be, but from our point of view you have to appreciate that this stroke is so extensive that she doesn't have the potential for rehabilitation. If she does arrest, she is going to suffer more injury and we could revive her but her quality of life would be zero."*

Always try to take a chaperone with you when you know a conversation is going to be difficult and you might run into trouble. Nurses are fantastic for this and, more often than not, have great relationships with relatives.

Katie, FY2 *"I had a high output family a couple of weeks ago. They had just lost their dad a few days before and then their mum had a massive stroke. She was only young, 62. She was in a really bad way and the consultant made the decision to DNAR. The family didn't want it, they didn't even want us to take bloods, yet they weren't willing for us to start on the end of life pathway either. They got angry and quite aggressive, so I said 'OK I think we need to stop', but they didn't listen. The senior nurse intervened and said 'Sorry but we can't have you shouting on the ward, there are other patients'. If you know you have a challenging family, you should have a chaperone."*

> **HERE ARE SOME TIPS FOR HANDLING DIFFICULT SITUATIONS:**
>
> - Explain the facts and be empathetic the whole way through.
> - Try to explore the bigger picture.
> - Check their understanding.
> - If relatives start getting too angry or confrontational simply excuse yourself and give them a minute to calm down. This can be a natural grief reaction.

How should I manage angry relatives?

Recognise that relatives may be angry because they are worried, frustrated, scared, anxious . . . . The list goes on. You should handle these situations by being *Safe, Slow, Low and Sympathetico!*

- **Safe**: bring a chaperone and make sure you know where the exit is.
- **Slow**: take everything slowly, let them vent before you speak, and slow down your speech as well as your body language to try and calm the situation.
- **Low**: keep the tone and pitch of your voice low.

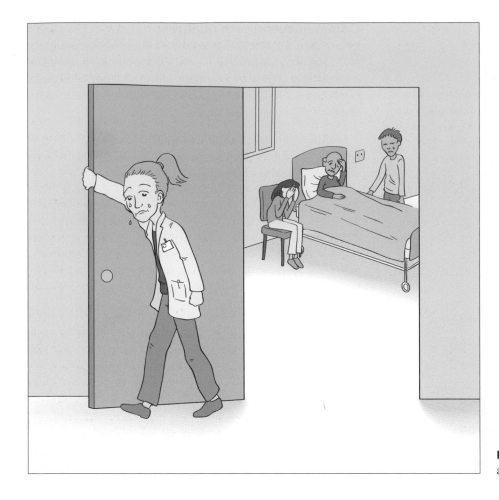

Figure 4.4 Seek out support if you've had a difficult conversation

• **Sympathetico**: state empathy obviously "*I can see that you are very angry*", offer an apology but don't impart blame "*I'm very sorry that this has happened*". Whatever you do DO NOT TELL THEM TO CALM DOWN, it will blow up in your face.

These situations are precisely the ones you should reflect on as it is highly likely you will have experienced such emotions yourself. Speak to a colleague about the events that unfolded. Most people find an angry person intimidating and may leave feeling a little 'shaken up'. Look after yourself so you can look after your patients; drifting around the ward an emotional wreck is no good to anyone (see Figure 4.4).

What if relatives want information about a patient you don't know?

This situation is tricky and could well happen if you are working in a small hospital where you are the only doctor on call. Often the nurses will bleep you because the family want to discuss their relative's care with a doctor. In this situation you might not know the patient and not be involved in their care. You then have to consider whether you are comfortable discussing the case in this manner with the relatives. If you do not feel it is appropriate – especially if bad news is involved – you must explain your reasons to the nurse as to why you cannot have that particular conversation. Also get the nurse to suggest to the family that they book an appointment with the patient's consultant the following day. It is better not to communicate at all than to communicate when you know little about the situation and may handle it badly. In this respect communication is all about the **TPP**: the appropriate **T**ime, **P**eople and **P**lace.

Breaking bad news

Breaking bad news is something that you should get practice doing with actors at medical school. You should be familiar with the process as you may be required to deliver bad news sooner than you think. That is not to say that you jump at the opportunity if presented. You must think carefully whether you have enough information about the patient before you decide to do it. Most importantly, take an experienced nurse with you. There are various mnemonics you can use for breaking bad news, SPIKES is particularly popular (Baille et al 2000).

• **Setting up the interview:** right place, bleep on silent to reduce interruptions etc.

• **Perception:** assess what the patient knows e.g. "what were our reasons for doing the colonoscopy?"

• **Invitation:** find out how much they want to know e.g. "how would you like the results?"

• **Knowledge:** this is where you fire a warning shot "unfortunately I have some bad news . . . " avoid using jargon and don't be blunt – patients will not appreciate you blurting out "I'm afraid you're going to die." Also, avoid using the phrase "there is nothing more we can do for you", as there is always something you can do: the whole palliative care pathway is designed to facilitate this.

- **Emotions and empathy:** this is the hardest part as it is often difficult to predict a patient's emotional reaction to bad news. There could be silence, crying, anger, denial . . . . Give them time to experience their emotions. Afterwards, address that emotion with empathy "I can see that . . . ".
- **Strategy and summary:** Having a clear plan reduces anxiety but make sure that the patient is ready to hear that plan. Close by checking understanding of what has been said.

This makes it sound simple, but, in reality, there are many personal barriers to breaking bad news. Rosen and Tesser (1970) described this charmingly as the MUM effect. The MUM (keeping Mum about Undesirable Messages) effect describes why it is so difficult to break bad news: the person delivering the bad news may feel anxious, burdened with the responsibility for delivering it, and fearful of a negative reaction. Unsurprisingly, this makes delivering bad news much harder, to the point where you become reluctant to deliver it. This effect intensifies when you perceive the patient to be distressed (Baille et al 2000).

Whilst you should understand that breaking bad news is not something typically done by an FY1, you may be the most appropriate person to break it if you have the best rapport with the patient. Each situation must be judged on its own merits, balancing the need for the patient to have the information in a timely manner against finding the best person to deliver it. Ultimately, the person delivering the bad news should always be certain of the information. Under no circumstances should you be delivering bad news on a 'suspected' or 'highly likely' premise. You MUST have all the accurate information and, if there are any doubts, wait for senior input. Conversely, you must NEVER deliver false hope; be honest and say you are unsure rather than reassuring the patient.

Carl, FY2 *"Although you may not be expected to do this, in reality, a lot of breaking bad news gets done on medical wards. You may be asked a direct question by a patient and you have to make a decision whether you are going to tell them that information or go and get help. If you feel comfortable and think it's the right thing for them to know, you can tell them. If it's not, then you need to find someone who will tell them in a timely manner. If they have asked for that information, they have a right to know but you have to balance this with the right person; there is nothing worse than a botched job of breaking bad news. Being quite personable and having a good rapport with patients will help. Make sure you get feedback afterwards though . . . ask a nurse to accompany you both as a witness and for support."*

Always consider whether you are the best person to break bad news. If it is not done properly, it can be disastrous and the patient and/or relatives will never forget. Here are a couple examples of breaking bad news badly, demonstrating how wrongly you can misinterpret the patient's views:

Daniel, Patient *"I was on the ward for kidney stones. I'd had a horrendous experience myself, so wasn't best pleased with the staff. The patient across from me had been very sick and, unfortunately, passed away during the night. They just drew the curtains around him and left the body in the bed! As if that wasn't bad enough, I heard the daughter come in the following morning and she walked straight past the reception into the ward. She was about to open the curtains when a nurse stopped her and said 'you can't go in there . . . he's dead!' I was shocked; I couldn't believe what had happened. That poor woman, she broke down in tears. I don't know whether they realised it was a relative of the patient but it was just horrific."*

Lorraine, ITU sister *"I use this as an example in training; it's one of the most horrendous things I've ever heard. The patient had sustained a massive head injury and had partial lobectomies. I went in with the consultant to speak to the wife and two sons, daughter, and in-laws. The consultant said 'your husband's operation was very successful. However, he will never be able to do anything for himself, never know who you are, never have a memory, or a personality . . . but his life will be normal longevity . . . . Can I make a suggestion'. The wife said 'Yes, please', and he said 'go home and make your family a lovely meal' and then he left! That was it. And I had to pick up the pieces . . . ."*

And a brilliant one to finish:

Lorraine, ITU sister *"There was one doctor particularly good at explaining it, he said: 'we have machines on ITU that can prolong life indefinitely.... But we are not prolonging your wife's life anymore; we are simply prolonging her inevitable death.' That worked very well."*

💡 **TOP 5 COMMUNICATION TIPS:**

1. Be sensitive towards patients, regardless of your mood.
2. Be meticulous about documentation, it is your legal lifeline.
3. Don't ignore disability, address it.
4. Dealing with relatives is an important part of patient care. Remember to be *Safe, Slow, Low and Sympathetico!*, and you'll handle difficult situations with ease.
5. Remember successful communication is all about **TPP**: the appropriate **T**ime, with the appropriate **P**eople, in the appropriate **P**lace.

5 Patient focus

Sarah, FY1 "*Part of patients getting better is them knowing and feeling they are are being well cared for and looked after.*"

Patient focus is all about making the care of your patient your first concern (GMC 2010). Foundation doctors are expected to:
- Gain trust from patients.
- Be empathetic, polite and courteous towards patients.
- Respect patient's wishes and work jointly towards their care.
- Build a relationship with both patients and their relatives.
- Consider patient safety at all times.

This means you will inevitably be required to deal with a wide range of problems concerning your patients. In this respect, foundation doctors are expected to:
- Demonstrate an ability to assimilate a range of information and identify key issues.
- Engage with wider issues and think creatively to solve problems and reach appropriate decisions.
- Be proactive, demonstrate initiative and attend to detail.

Being the best for your patients

TOP TIPS ON BEING THE BEST FOR YOUR PATIENTS:

- **Talk *to* your patients, not about them**

Julia, ST2 "*When on a ward round, try not to talk about patients in front of them – address them. If you hear your consultant saying for example 'this patient is two days post lap-choli . . . ' try to steer them away from doing it. Ask the patient how they are doing and always go back and talk to them afterwards if you feel they've been left in the dark.*"

- **Look after yourself so you can best care for your patients** (see Figure 5.1)

Bill, Patient "*Look after your own health – sometimes I am looking at the doctor and they're so ill I'm thinking 'Should they really be here? . . . They look worse than I do'. It does make you question whether they can do their job properly.*"

- **Realise that patients are your customers . . . they are always right!** Be mindful that patients are people with lives outside the hospital. Your job is to get them out of that bed and back to the real world as soon as you can.

Charlotte, Consultant Surgeon "*Really good doctors don't care about the boundaries of care and see patients as human beings rather than 'that's not my speciality so I'm not doing it'. I was seeing a patient transferred from dermatology with really bad leg ulcers who required urgent investigations. The junior* said 'eugh . . . why do we have to look after that patient from dermatology?' That attitude of 'someone else's patient not mine' is simply not tolerated. I was really not impressed.*"

- **Be empathetic.** This means understanding where the patient is coming from and that means working out what they are thinking. Without empathy you may fall into a trap: adopting a defensive position, or simply missing the mark altogether.

Tony, Consultant Surgeon "*Sometimes it can take an hour of conversation to develop a rapport with a patient so they trust you enough to let you treat them. I remember one chap seeming very angry with us, but in fact I had read it all wrong – he was just very anxious and fighting his feelings. I handled it fine but I would read that differently again.*"

- **ALWAYS examine your patient.** A clinical error such as this is inexcusable.

Shan, Consultant Surgeon "*I know plenty of law suits because the clinician has failed to examine. A colleague of mine came to see me about a breast lump . . . she said, 'of all the surgeons in this hospital, you're the first one to treat me like a patient and actually examine me.' I thought this was remarkable, and wholly unacceptable.*"

- **Know your responsibility for social care as much as medical care.** This is because social factors have a huge effect on the patient's physical and mental health and will determine whether they return to hospital or not. Although the nursing staff will largely liaise with OTs, physios and social services, you need to appreciate social discharge from the point of view of:
  - Which patients require social input.
  - How their social requirements are assessed.
  - The support they will receive at home.
  - Being able to report back to the patient information about their social placement.
- **Don't forget about families and relatives and be conscious that you are always being critiqued.** Most complaints come from how you present yourself to others rather than the patient.
- **Be meticulous about your clinical style** and never underestimate the need to be conscientious and diligent. This may require occasionally going the extra mile to facilitate the best patient care.

Patient advocacy

Sunita, FY1 "*If the patient thinks that your consultant is doing a bad job then you have to relay that information. . . . You have to just stand back from the fact it's your senior and be the patient's advocate.*"

Advocacy is again something that is often discussed, but, in reality, it is difficult to perceive its relationship with everyday

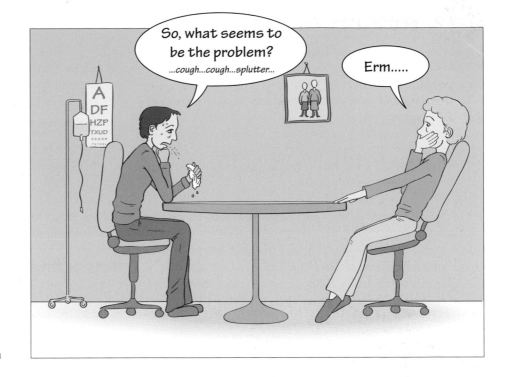

Figure 5.1 As a doctor you have a responsibility to look after your own health

practice. Basically, it means fighting someone else's corner using your own unique knowledge base and skill set. Whilst there are external services for this such as the Patient Advice and Liaison Service (PALS 2009) – you must also remember that you are an advocate for your patient when it comes to their care. As the junior member on your team, you will have the largest proportion of contact with your patients, aside from the nurses. This means you have to understand where the patient is coming from and stand back from any difficult behaviour or negative opinions about your colleagues.

Samyami, FY2 *"I was working on a surgical ward with a patient in hospital for appendicitis. He also had long-standing hyperkalaemia and when he came in his potassium was 7.0. I was working nights when he became symptomatic; I treated him and he was fine by the morning, but his potassium remained high. My team didn't think this was a priority, and, given his surgical problem was fixed, felt he should be allowed to go home. I spoke up as I didn't feel he was fit for discharge. The nurse specialist was adamant nothing was wrong, so the consultant heard us both out. The consultant agreed that I could investigate because I wasn't happy with it. My team didn't like it as it delayed his discharge for two days whilst I went on a detective hunt to find out what was wrong. In the end it turned out he was taking steroids and needed sodium replacement. I don't regret it, and I would do the same again if my patient needed it."*

This case highlights the fact that the appropriate action for medical professionals – regardless of position – is to raise concerns about patient safety. The GMC (2012) recently adapted such guidance to ensure that a culture of openness is more fruitfully embraced. As a doctor, you are expected to speak up if you think care is being compromised by anything: staff, procedures or policies. You should not hesitate to report a concern and the GMC (2012) explain why:

- Your duty to put patients first overrides everything else.
- You are protected by law against being victimised or dismissed for exposing malpractice.
- Reasonable belief is enough justification, not hard proof.
- You are not in the position to put it right yourself.

However, you must do this by following the appropriate procedure and going through the proper channels. The correct reporting procedures are detailed below. However, it is advisable to consult your local trust policy when you start your job.

For adverse events or near misses:
- Fill in a CAE or critical incident form to prevent future recurrence.
- Usually these are not escalated beyond your team.

Jackie, ST1 *"The nurses won't think twice about doing a CAE form; they are clued up on good practice. They did one for me when I was working on a post-natal ward at the weekend. There were loads of baby checks to be done, and I kept getting called to deliveries. I couldn't get through all the checks by the time I left at 9 p.m. and the poor night SHO was discharging until 2 a.m.! You can't avoid going to an emergency C-section though. This was a staffing issue . . . if you don't fill in a form, nothing will change."*

For serious incidents or repeated adverse events that are not being adequately addressed:

• Raise the issue with your consultant.
• Then raise it with your educational supervisor or foundation director.
• Keep a record of your concerns and the steps taken to deal with the situation.
• Make sure the patient receives both an explanation and an apology.

If you have no joy internally, or feel the matter has been dealt with unsatisfactorily, then you can:

• Raise the issue with the GMC.
• Make your concern public – providing that you do not breach confidentiality.

It is highly likely that you will have to report bad practice at some point in your career. The irony is that you are more likely to notice it as a foundation doctor as, new to the system – there is less propensity for adopting the "this is how we do it here" mentality.

Charlotte, FY2 *"I had an experience of being constantly undermined by a senior nurse. All my colleagues felt the same way . . . it wasn't an isolated thing. It went so far that she was making me prescribe a drug that I wasn't familiar with – I was unsure of the dose and she wouldn't allow me to check it. That was the last straw. I realised then that it wasn't safe for me or the patient. When you have serious concerns like that it needs to be raised to the supervisor and if not them, your foundation director or FY1 mentor. I raised my concerns with my supervisor rather than the nurse in this instance. They were very supportive but this person was a stable member of the team and very little could be done. Consequently I raised it externally on a deanery visit and they dealt with it, so whistle-blowing is not a bad thing – you need to protect yourself and your patients."*

If you are ever unsure of what to do GMC guidance (2012) suggests:

• Asking a senior or impartial colleague for advice.
• Contacting your medical defence body or professional association such as the BMA.
• Contacting the GMC for confidential advice.
• Contacting 'Public Concern at Work': a charity which provides free, confidential legal advice.

When does crossing the line become a 'Fitness to Practise' (FTP) issue?

By definition FTP involves "*serious or persistent failures*" and therefore gross misconduct. This includes situations such as those involving (GMC 2006):

• Risk of harm that cannot be dealt with locally.
• Deliberate or reckless misconduct.
• A health problem where the doctor refuses to follow medical advice and poses a continued risk to patients.
• A doctor abusing patients' trust or violating their autonomy.

This may be something that you flag up, but will never be a matter that you yourself should deal with. You should report such concerns to your educational supervisor, foundation clinical lead or foundation programme director. They will escalate the matter to the deanery board for 'Doctors in Difficulty' and then to the GMC if necessary (see Chapter 6).

Tim, Foundation Programme Director *"The only incident I've heard of – on the grapevine – of an FY1 being struck off was a heroin addict who was being abusive towards patients. Drink driving for example would be a 'Doctors in Difficulty' issue. Most of these can be resolved with support – and maybe an extra year's training if necessary. Many go on to be fantastic doctors, even if they do have a rough start."*

Respecting personal beliefs

Under no circumstances should you impose your personal beliefs on patients unless they are directly relevant to their care. However, this can be tricky as you may not realise you have an issue with something until it suddenly hits you square in the face. For that reason you need to stay alert to how your own personal beliefs could interfere with care. If this happens, you must explain this to the patient as well as their right to seek treatment elsewhere (GMC 2008b). Two situations to be aware of involving strong personal beliefs include the refusal of blood products by a Jehovah's Witness and the circumcision of male children for non-medical purposes. Jehovah's Witnesses are discussed below.

HERE ARE A FEW TIPS FOR SITUATIONS INVOLVING PATIENTS WHO ARE JEHOVAH'S WITNESSES:

• If you have a patient who is a Jehovah's Witness, don't assume they will automatically refuse blood products.
• Enquire about their views and answer questions with honesty and respect.
• Seek senior advice and consult the local hospital guidelines about the options available.
• Some patients may not be aware of the different blood products and which are deemed acceptable or not. If you need further advice, then, with the patient's consent, you can contact the local Hospital Liaison Committee (HLC). They should have a helpline set up by the Watchtower Society (Jehovah's Witness society), which is available via the 24-hour Hospital Information Service.
• "Bloodless medical procedures" are available in some hospitals. Again, you can get these details from the HLC (GMC 2008b).

Jackie, ST1 *"We had a patient in his late teens admitted under surgery with a splenic rupture. He initially went to one hospital and was then transferred to ours because we had cell salvage facilities. He didn't have any problems in theatre but there was a fairly high risk he would need transfusion. You always try to accommodate patient's wishes as best as possible."*

Tricky decisions involving treatment: consent without capacity

All patients with capacity are assumed able to consent to treatment. Patients also have the right to refuse medical care (if over 18 years), even if it means they may die. This premise is complicated whenever a patient lacks the ability to consent. Broadly speaking, you will encounter three different types of situations where you may be required to treat a patient without their consent:
- **Psychiatric**: e.g. a patient with acute onset psychosis could be treated under the Mental Health Act (MHA).
- **Organic:** e.g. a patient with delirium tremens could be treated under the Mental Capacity Act (MCA) 2005.
- **Emergencies:** e.g. a patient with diabetic ketoacidosis (DKA) could be treated under the doctrine of necessity.

The MHA, MCA and doctrine of necessity are generally very well covered in medical school. Moreover, the MHA should be fairly self-explanatory for a given psychiatric case and not something that you would be involved in as a junior. What is most relevant to FY1 practice is how to approach organic concerns of impaired capacity.

If a patient lacks the capacity to decide you should firstly (GMC 2010):
- Know what decisions about care are to be made.
- Check through all the notes for any legal documentation concerning care, e.g. advanced directives.

Next you should enquire about a legal proxy e.g. lasting power of attorney or court-appointed-deputy (England and Wales). This is because, if there is no legal proxy, your consultant – as the patient's doctor – would be responsible for the decisions made about treatment for that patient. This means deciding on the "overall benefit" of treatment. In this situation you must involve those close to the patient as well as other members of the healthcare team to help inform your decision. Do not despair if there are no close family or friends available. In this instance, you can contact an IMCA – as Nick did for the patient who couldn't communicate (see Chapter 4, p. 38).

An IMCA can be consulted in most difficult decision-making processes; including where there may be a conflict of interest. They act as an independent person outside of the healthcare system to represent the patient's views. Their service may also be required where relatives or friends are available but one of the following circumstances applies (Lee 2007):
- The friends and relatives are unwilling to be consulted about the patient's best interests.
- They are too frail to be consulted.
- They are too far away to logistically be consulted.
- They refuse.
- You suspect abuse in the relationship.

Places you can look to contact this service include the Department of Health (DH) website, PALS or the Citizens Advice Bureau (CAB). This however does not apply when an urgent decision needs to be made, as in an emergency.

In a life or death situation you treat under the doctrine of necessity. Here, if the consultant "reasonably believes" a treatment is necessary to save the patient's life and the patient lacks capacity, then the treatment can be given without a formal assessment. This is because in an emergency – for example, when a patient is having a cardiac arrest – it is not really appropriate to be filling in paperwork. You would, of course, do your best to keep the patient informed and consulted where possible (DCA 2005).

Most importantly, wherever your job is, your trust will have local policy documents on capacity and consent. Familiarise yourself with them when you start; or at least know how and where to access them.

What about confidentiality and information-sharing?

You will often find that those close to the patient will want information about the patient's diagnosis and the likely progression of the course of the illness. If the patient has capacity, you must get their permission before sharing this information. If they lack capacity, it is reasonable to assume that (unless otherwise indicated) they would want those closest to them informed about such information (GMC 2010). Remember that if the patient expressly wishes their relatives not to be involved – you must respect this – even after death.

Matthew, GP *"We had an interesting case recently of a patient who didn't want her information divulged to her mum even after death. This patient had many complex alcohol and mental health issues and she didn't want any of that divulged. The mum is trying to go through the ombudsman and everything to get it. You do find that comes up quite commonly but ultimately you have to respect the patient's wishes."*

Can those close to the patient make the overall decision?

Only if they are legally appointed to do so and this is formalised as such. A patient can nominate someone to be kept informed and consulted about treatment, but this does not mean they have legal guardianship to make the final decision. You should be explicit about this when discussing such issues and make it clear that their role is advisory rather than definitive. If a patient wishes to nominate someone to make decisions on their behalf for a given situation (i.e. if they lose capacity), they need to formalise it legally (GMC 2010).

End of Life care

Matthew, GP *"One challenging factor starting as a junior stems from the realisation that people do actually die in your care, and it's not something you realise until it actually happens. The first few times it really affects you . . . and you might not think it will . . . until it actually does."*

The End of Life (EOL) pathway includes any patient likely to die within the next twelve months. As a junior you will, in part, be expected to put patients on the EOL pathway. Prepare for situations which may require you to complete the appropriate paperwork. Moreover, if you are having difficulties dealing with something or feel uncomfortable, seek support from your colleagues rather than burying your head in the sand.

🗣 **Sophie, FY1** *"Putting a patient onto the EOL pathway is something I've had to do . . . and was very uncomfortable doing. My registrar made the decision, and I completed the paperwork. I asked the ward sister to check what I had written and she agreed with what I had done, but I definitely felt underprepared for this."*

Although not expected to make EOL decisions as a foundation doctor, you should understand the reasons for starting the EOL pathway as well as the process. Be aware that the risks and benefits of each treatment are not always clear cut. What you aim to avoid is causing the patient further undue stress or prolongation of the dying process, and this should be communicated to close friends and family where appropriate (GMC 2010).

The GMC (2010) outlines the EOL decision-making process as follows:
1. The doctor and patient make an assessment of the patient's condition, which will include medical history, views, experience and knowledge.
2. The specialist registrar/consultant combines their experience and knowledge with the patient's opinion about their condition (where possible) to identify the relevant options. The options should then be explained to the patient with the benefits, burdens and risks of each one. The doctor may recommend one, but they must not pressure the patient into accepting their advice.
3. The patient makes the decision – regardless of the doctor's opinion.
4. The same process applies when a legal proxy is appointed to make the decision, whilst trying to include the patient as far as is possible.

What about a DNAR (Do Not Attempt Resuscitation) decision?
Interestingly, a patient does not have to be informed about this. If a patient is at foreseeable risk of cardiac or respiratory arrest, and the consultant decides that resuscitation would not be successful, then they should consider carefully whether to tell the patient. This decision is never assumed and it is likely that, as a clinician with the closest relationship with the patient, it will be your responsibility to explore whether they would wish to know about the DNAR. If they decline, seek permission to share this information with others such as a family member. If they lack capacity, the decision should be shared appropriately but ultimately, signing the DNAR is the lead clinician's call (GMC 2010).

You must remember to always record any discussions and reasoning in the patient's records as this will be your responsibility. Furthermore, the EOL pathway, particularly the decision

to DNAR, can be difficult for relatives to come to terms with. Recognise this and be sympathetic. Imagine if your family member was in that position, how would you feel?

🗣 **Samyami, FY2** *"Clinically making a decision not to resuscitate can be hard for relatives and they can get very angry: in their eyes you're giving up on treatment, you don't care and you're leaving them to die. I have seen it so many times on the ward. You can put your best effort into explaining it, but they usually stop listening to you. At the end of the day, you have to remember that the lead clinician has responsibility for deciding overall benefit even if the family disagree. Conversely, it can happen when the patient is started on the EOL pathway too late. Those well-read on dignity and dying will question it and would have liked it earlier; 'you made my mum suffer for two weeks instead of one' – relatives can be angry at that as well."*

Difficult patients

It is impossible to gel with all your patients. Here are some tips in dealing with patients with difficult behaviours:
• **Be prepared to experience a multitude of emotions**.

🗣 **Michael, GP** *"As a junior you are flooded with many emotions you will not have experienced before. You end up having to deal with a lot of people who are very emotional, angry and upset. Most of the time this is a natural response to the situation they are in . . . handling this is very tricky as a junior. Ensure that you have had some good communication skills training and recognise that empathy and understanding are very important. You will always have the odd occasion where relatives may pin you down to talk to you about difficult issues such as end of life care. Work out how to deal with certain types of emotion."*

• **Recognise difficult behaviour may be a defence mechanism**.

🗣 **Terry, Consultant Surgeon** *"Patients may be belligerent and rude and walking away from the ward rather than to theatre . . . that becomes particularly challenging to manage . . . sometimes it's just because they have a hospital phobia, so you really have to understand where they are coming from."*

• **Never raise your voice or get into an argument with a patient. If the situation is too heavy, politely excuse yourself.**

🗣 **Carl, FY2** *"On call I went to see a patient with chronic back problems. He had been in multiple times under the neurosurgeons. Despite being on many different analgesics, he was still in acute pain and asking for IV Morphine. The pain team reviewed his case and said he didn't need it. It was 8 p.m. before I went to see him. The nursing staff told me that in-between his IV Morphine he was going outside for a fag. He was very difficult and very aggressive straight away:*

demanding IV Morphine. I told him that the pain team had reviewed his case and that I could only give him Oromorph. At which point he got up and started remonstrating . . . threatening to go to the papers. I repeated that I couldn't offer him anything more overnight, and the pain team would see him in the morning. The patient then started screaming at me again, so I politely left and went to document everything. Half an hour later the nursing staff said he wanted to apologise. Being firm and walking away when I realised I wasn't going to get anywhere worked; when a patient is angry, you need to be diplomatic and reasoned. Before you go to see the patient, think about your options and don't give in just because they are shouting. If it is getting out of hand you should try to end the conversation reasonably."

• **Support your colleagues when they have difficult patients. Respect that if they come to you with a difficult patient, it's for a good reason**.

Matthew, GP *"Nurses do a very good job and protect a lot of staff. When you are asked to sort out an angry patient, it's a big deal. Likewise, if you get a call at night for a patient who is agitated and wandering, the nurses will have tried everything in their locker of imagination as to how they can deal with it. They won't call you for nothing and that's hard to appreciate at first – they deal with an awful lot of stuff you just never see."*

TOP 5 TIPS ON PATIENT FOCUS:

1. Lead by example.
2. Always make sure the patient is your first priority.
3. Don't be afraid to highlight bad practice.
4. Check who the patient wants to be involved in their treatment.
5. Be mindful of your own safety and leave if the situation gets too heated.

Nicola, FY1 *"Make it known you are keen to be a team member. . . . Don't just turn up, do your job and go home. If you want to have a career, that's inadvisable."*

A foundation doctor who is a good team-player is expected to:
• Have the capability and willingness to work effectively with others.
• Be helpful to others, collaborative, and respectful of others' views.
• Offer support and advice.
• Share tasks appropriately.
• Understand their own and others' roles within the team.
• Consult with others where appropriate.

Understanding teamwork

Carl, FY2 *"Teamwork is all about being adaptable. As a medical student you come from a background where you structure your own work and all responsibility is up to you. Suddenly, you are in a team where you cannot simply work on your own; you have to communicate well with everyone. Even if their way of working is completely alien to yours, you have to find a way around it. That's not always the easiest thing to do."*

Besides considering your personality type (see Chapter 1), an additional way of understanding yourself is by looking at the part you play in a team. Teamwork is vital to your job as an FY1, and one of the specific aspects covered by the SJT. A great deal of research has been done on the effective functioning of teams and the different roles that team members take in order to aid successful teamwork. The best-known model of team descriptors is Belbin's Team Roles (Belbin 2010a [first published 1993]). If you find it hard to identify the roles you prefer to adopt, try a formal questionnaire online to help you (see www.belbin.com).

Belbin's Team Roles measure behaviour, not personality. People gravitate towards the roles which suit their natural style, but where team members seek to take on similar functions, some may adapt to take on other roles. No one role is better than another; they all play a component part in the overall team performance. A really effective team will display a balance in the Team Roles being performed; too much of one behaviour or the absence of another can throw a team into disarray.

Understanding the different Team Roles will help you to think more clearly about your individual contribution to a team and how other people's contributions are different, but equally valid. You may be able to use this insight to spot the problems when teamwork breaks down: a consistent theme in the SJT. You can then share the problem with the team or, if necessary, adapt your behaviour to improve the situation.

Belbin's Team Roles

Annie, Consultant *"Every member of a team in a hospital has to have their role defined . . . if they're not defined, you start having conflict."*

Belbin (2010b [first published 1981]) describes nine Team Roles. Each Team Role has strengths and corresponding "allowable" weaknesses. These are described below, coupled with some advice for a person who takes on this particular role:

1. **Plant:** Whilst a natural problem-solver, creative and imaginative, the plant tends to ignore incidentals: *remember to fill in a Clinically Adverse Event (CAE) form, even for near misses!*

2. **Resource Investigator (RI):** Enthusiastic and outgoing, the RI creates networks outside the team but quickly loses momentum once the first flush of enthusiasm for a project/idea is over: *remember to stay focused – even if your new rotation has lost its charm after a few weeks.*

3. **Monitor Evaluator:** Evaluates what others present, judges and weighs up the options. Unfortunately though, this can make the monitor evaluator overly critical of others: *remember to give constructive rather than critical feedback when teaching medical students.*

4. **Coordinator:** Spots other people's talents and delegates accordingly, but this can result in coordinators avoiding their own share of the work: *remember that teamwork is a two-way process – if you give bloods to the nurses, you can help them out with a catheter or two later on.*

5. **Implementer:** Keeps it practical and turns ideas into tasks that need to be done. However, the Implementer can be inflexible and slow to respond: *prioritise and reprioritise jobs according to their urgency; if you feel you struggle with flexibility, ask for help.*

6. **Completer Finisher (CF):** Whilst painstakingly meticulous, seeing things through to the end, the CF worries unnecessarily and doesn't like to hand over to others: *if you find yourself waking at midnight wondering if you handed over that investigation, it's okay to ring the ward and check . . . just don't make a habit of it.*

7. Teamworker: Cooperative and diplomatic, the Team-worker brings people together harmoniously, but can be swayed too much by others' opinions: *advice from the nursing staff is invaluable, but remember, at the end of the day, the buck stops with your decision.*

8. Shaper: Enjoys the pressure of delivering to a deadline. The Shaper is dynamic and driven but can put others' backs up by being over-zealous: *when diving in with your A to E approach, don't forget your manners!*

9. Specialist: Contributes valuable expertise and knowledge from a narrow field, but can be unable to see things from a wider perspective: *your nurse specialist can help you out with everything from pain management to stoma care but overall, your consultant sees things more holistically.*

Michael, GP *"A key thing to understand is what your role is in the whole team. Sometimes you are dumped on as a junior so it's recognising:* 'do I have to do the bloods, do I have to do the venflons?' *It's about knowing what you're responsible for, but realising that you are part of a team. On the other hand, it may be that you are the only person there that can do that job at that particular time so sometimes you might have to do tasks that you don't consider part of your remit."*

Team Role Descriptors and icons reproduced by kind permission of BELBIN, UK – www.belbin.com

Understanding your role

Sunita, FY2 *"If you're prepared to work a little bit harder it makes things easier and you'll be a better team member."*

Having considered the theoretical dimensions of a team, here are some practical tips:
• Never shy away from asking for help. At the end of the day, there is a person at the end of the phone – not a monster!
• Teamwork is about give and take. Don't take the attitude "that's not my job". If you help a team member out, they will be there to help you when you need it. Good teamwork will lessen your workload and lighten your day.
• Learn to delegate. Sometimes you are dumped on, so know what tasks you can allocate to others during these times.
• Divide jobs evenly amongst the juniors so everyone does their fair share.
• Every hospital works in a slightly different way, find this out from the outset.
• Understand that your role is CLINICAL not theoretical: bloods, cannulas, TTOs and recognising ill patients are your bread and butter.

Samyami, FY2 *"What's important to understand is that 80% of the work you do in med school is theoretical. On the wards it's about practical skills, being sensible, organised and writing things down properly. That transition between balancing theoretical and practical knowledge is key. If you're not confident in your clinical practical skills then carrying out the first steps of management – no matter how good your theoretical knowledge is – becomes very difficult to execute."*

Sometimes, you may find yourself going above and beyond the standard duty of care. This is because you are human as well as being a doctor. Your sense of humanity is what makes you a great doctor. Nevertheless, be careful of going beyond the boundaries too often, as you may find you sacrifice your own well-being in the process. Learn to balance your needs with those of your colleagues and your patients.

Faraz, FY1 *"Some patients you have stronger relationships with. I had a patient on surgery that I had been looking after for a couple of months. Despite optimum treatment we knew he was going to die, and I was on call. He didn't have any family close by and he wanted someone to talk to and hold his hand. I had to juggle priorities of being the only FY1 on call and being with this man in his last minutes. I decided to stay with him and answer any bleeps as they came rather than talk to the nursing staff or have a break as I would usually do if it's quiet. I spent most of that night with him just so he wasn't alone in his last minutes . . . even though you get used to death, it's never easy."*

At the end of the day, if you feel you are doing too much, you probably are. Recognise your limitations and speak up. It could be that your rotation is not well enough staffed, and others before have had similar problems:

Eve, FY2 *"Workload can be very variable. A team may not be well staffed or may have a workload beyond their resources, so you end up staying well beyond 5 p.m. whilst your friends are going home on time in their job. I stayed 1–2 hours beyond 5 p.m. every day for the first 2 months on my first rotation. Part of this was learning the job and getting quicker, but the other part was not knowing what was an unreasonable workload. You need to take stock and think whether it is reasonable to expect you to work that number of hours beyond what you are being paid for and what is reasonable in terms of your health and general well-being. If you feel you are struggling, you need to raise it with your educational supervisor. There is no shame in saying you are struggling, as chances are the previous house officers were, and the next one will be. There are some jobs where workload is way beyond staffing and, unless you raise it, it will never change. You can also ask for your hours to be monitored if you think it's particularly unfair. Some people have done that and their FY1 jobs have changed . . . one of the ones I did now has 2 juniors rather than 1."*

What are the pitfalls which cause teamwork to break down?

- Not being reliable; avoiding doing outpatient clinic letters for 3–4 weeks.
- Being bleeped and not answering.
- Being abrupt with colleagues – especially with secretaries.
- Being defensive.
- Blaming others for mistakes.
- Not completing paperwork appropriately.
- Not writing legibly.
- Not being accurate and making things up!

Christine, Consultant *"As an FY1 you have to be approachable and nice and be able to speak to other disciplines. If we get a secretary – or a nurse – coming to tell us that an FY1 doctor was rude, we don't want the headache of managing that conflict. Being pleasant is a very important quality."*

What are the consequences of these pitfalls?

Jeff, Consultant *"Not being accurate is annoying and we see that a lot. If you are not accurate with the doses of medication when taking a history and don't cross-check the dose and the letter goes to the GP, the GP comes back and says 'I'm sorry the dose you sent me is incorrect.' That creates extra work for me. First, I have to get the records out – which might mean trawling through the 400 to 500 patients on my workload. I then have to fish out the records to look at the last consultation and look at what was written. If the handwriting isn't clear, it makes it even more difficult. Then I have to call the patient and ask what medications they are on, go to the pharmacy and look at the prescription, fax a letter to the GP – all that because the junior wasn't accurate. . . . See how much work is created if things aren't checked properly."*

Effective handovers

Fraz, FY1 *"If you request bloods, X-rays, scans and then go home and forget to check them or hand them over, you will find yourself waking up at 2 a.m. But you have to ring the on-call and get them to check: regardless of the time. Always be aware that if you request them, they are your responsibility."*

Handovers are vital for maintaining patient care whilst you are off duty. You cannot simply leave at the end of your shift without making sure that care is safeguarded (GMC 2009a). The aim is to reach a shared understanding amongst staff about the priorities for each patient (BMA 2004b).

THE ROYAL COLLEGE OF SURGEONS (RCS 2007) AND THE BRITISH MEDICAL ASSOCIATION (BMA 2004B) OFFER THE FOLLOWING TIPS FOR A SAFE HANDOVER:

1. **Set the scene.**
   - Set sufficient time aside within working hours, in a quiet area: ideally the same time every day.
   - Keep it a "bleep free" zone.
   - The most senior clinician should set out a brief plan.
   - Have access to lab results, X-rays, clinical information, the intranet/internet and telephones.
   - Structure the team discussion so only one person speaks at a time.
   - Encourage a culture where information is challenged: there are no 'stupid' questions.
2. **Minimum requirements.**
   - Patient's FULL name and date of birth.
   - Date patient was admitted to hospital.
   - Where the patient is (ward and bed).
   - Current diagnosis.
   - Results of any significant investigations.
   - Outstanding tasks, e.g. chasing investigations, bloods etc.
3. **Additional information.**
   - Patient condition, e.g. stable, sick – MEWS (Modified Early Warning Score) if used.
   - Urgency of review – Now? 1 hour? None?
   - Management plan including "what to do if . . . " contingency plan.
   - Operational issues e.g. ITU beds available? Discharge planning.

What are the common difficulties compromising a handover?

- Including "non-essential" information means you can't see the wood for the trees.
- Not including enough information means the patient gets put to the bottom of the pile.
- Not having a checklist of information to hand over means things get missed.
- Not having the information handed over in writing: you cannot possibly remember everything.
- Speaking over one another such that information gets lost and misinterpreted.

Craig, FY2 *"Every shift works better with effective handovers. We work shorter shifts now, so there are more handovers. Each time a different doctor takes on the information, so, unless it's clear what jobs you want doing, it becomes like Chinese whispers. By the third handover someone has the patient's details and something about abdo pain but they don't have a clue what they are supposed to be doing. The worst part is that, if you don't have the information, and you are busy, that's going to be a low priority as you can always say 'well,* we didn't know'. *If you have ten patients you know aren't very well, you are not going to concentrate your time on the one you don't know anything about!"*

A colleague phones to say they are running late. They cannot give you a definite time they will be there and you have made dinner plans. How should you proceed?
Patient safety is paramount, and therefore you should take steps to see that the handover is achieved in a suitable manner so that you can get away: you are not expected to stay hours beyond the end of your shift. The handover should be to a colleague working on the ward – most likely a registrar. This is not a responsibility you can delegate to a nurse, and it would be unfair to do so. Moreover, communication must be in verbal as well as written form, as you cannot rely on your colleague coming onto shift to prioritise patients simply on the basis of the notes. It is time consuming to fumble through notes attempting to find previous management plans. This could delay review and potentially compromise patient safety. Be proactive and make sure your senior has all the information (ISFP 2012).

Understanding your colleagues' roles
Although there are a multitude of team members, the nursing team, your consultant, and the radiology department are the ones discussed here. You might like to consider others' roles whilst on your clinical placements. Take five minutes out of your day to have a chat with the ward clerks, the porters, the laboratory staff – anyone whose roles and responsibilities you are not certain of – and consider their relationship to the running of the hospital.

The nursing team
Undoubtedly you will have heard that you should cherish the nursing team: they are your best friends. Here are some reasons why nurses are invaluable:
- **They can show you where everything is.**

Nick, FY1 *"My first shifts at this hospital were night shifts and it was quite daunting as it was a new job, new hospital and I didn't know any of the patients at all. I didn't even know how to request bloods, and when you're on nights there are no seniors – well there are, but you only call them if it's serious, not to ask how to request bloods! The nursing staff definitely saved me on my first three nights: showed me everything. They're your best friends when you start I would say, they really are."*

- **They can give you advice on management.**

Sarah, FY1 *"Listen to the nursing staff – they do know what they are talking about. If circumstances arise where the opinion is not mutual, I explain why, so we come up with a shared understanding. Realistically, I accept advice from nurses every day. When you first start you feel like you are constantly demanding things off them – almost to the point of feeling like a nag – but as you develop your relationship you realise there's so much give and take."*

- **They are closest to the patients and their relatives, and can raise their concerns to you.**

Des, Psychiatric Nurse *"Nurses are at the bedside with the patient and the relatives see that. You build up a strong relationship surprisingly quickly. Nurses are also there for the emotional support of the family as well as the patient. We have an intimate relationship with patients; we can spot unusual things, as well as raise things that they haven't told you. That information is crucial for medics to have if they want communication to be successful."*

Above all, however, you must remember to communicate what you need in order for your relationship to blossom – nurses may be fantastic, but they are not mind readers:

Tim, FY1 *"It's really important to tell the nurses what you want done. If you just write in the notes and then leave, no one will know. I was wondering for the first week why my plans weren't getting through quickly – it was only because I was being an idiot and didn't realise that I was supposed to tell the nurses. It's really stupid and obvious now, but I learned this pretty quickly!"*

Besides helping the juniors, nurses have a vital relationship with patients. You should remember two things in this respect:
1. Nurses will stop at nothing to advocate the best for their patients. So if you don't respond to their request and they feel their patient is compromised, they will have no problems ringing your consultant at home, in the middle of the night (see Figure 6.1).

Des, Psychiatric Nurse *"One of the patients on the ward was complaining of a cold leg. We called the consultant who bluntly told us to put a sock on her leg and he would be back in the morning to check on it. We weren't happy with this so eventually we rang a different doctor for another opinion. An hour later she was seen – her leg had gone completely white – and she was rushed to the main hospital for a DVT. If we hadn't been so vigilant and been willing to get a second opinion, she would have lost her leg."*

2. Nurses are the guardians of safety.

Lorraine, ITU Sister *"As a nurse you find you are watching what everyone else is doing to safeguard the patient. It doesn't matter what level the person is, there is always potential for dangerous practice, so that is added pressure. I remember one incident of a patient who was seriously ill with a severe head injury. He needed some drug therapy to stop him fitting, so the nurses drew the drugs up. The doctor then came in, picked up the syringe and injected it into an arterial line by mistake! This caused massive problems. The patient survived – despite a necrotic arm – and it went to court. That was someone not knowing the difference between an arterial line and a peripheral cannula. It made you realise you have to*

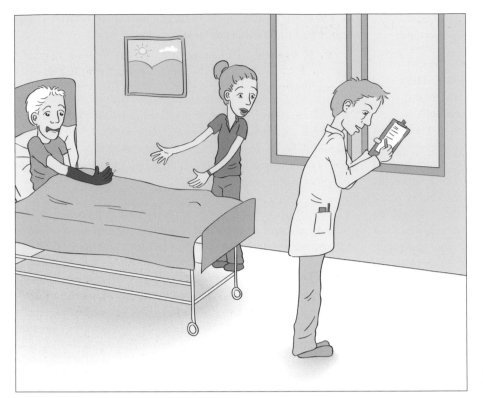

Figure 6.1 Listen to the nurses: they also have the patients' best interests at heart

have eyes in the back of your head. When there are a lot of people in a critical environment like that, there is added pressure on us to safeguard the patient and watch what everyone else is doing – particularly as they may not be familiar with the equipment."

Nurses also have the added pressures of:
• Long days, long shifts and few breaks with stretched resources.
• Dealing with anxious relatives wanting lots of information, combating angry relatives, handling wandering patients.
• Delivering the prescribed drugs at the right time.
• Getting patients discharged.

Jennifer, Nurse *"Nursing is about bringing together everyone to make it safe. We try to achieve what the medics want us to achieve, in a safe manner, whilst watching and keeping everyone else safe as well. We should spot if you are about to make a mistake as we have more experience."*

The consultant

Having been on the wards, have you ever really considered the responsibilities that your consultant has? Here are a few pressures to appreciate:
• Busy workload: ward rounds, clinics, theatre, paperwork, etc.
• Politics of the job: staffing, resources, funding, budgets, salary and pension changes, etc.

• Duty to communicate with colleagues – especially with GPs.
• Responding to phone calls and emails.
• Ultimate responsibility for ALL their patients.
• Training and personal development for themselves and their staff.

Mithun, Consultant Psychiatrist *"Responsibility ends with me; if something a junior does is wrong, it goes to the consultant. My job doesn't end with the day. Juniors and SHOs can finish, but, if my job doesn't get done right, there is no-one to take it off my back. Juniors also need to understand that, at the end of the day, my priorities are to the patient. You must give us time and plan ahead; I don't want the junior coming to me wanting training expecting me to drop everything. I have a long-term relationship with my patients and I must be sensitive to their needs above all else. Juniors leave but my patients stay with me, it is important to remember this."*

The radiology department

Negotiating a scan for your patients is something that you will have to do week in and week out. What you have to realise is that radiographers and radiologists also have a list of things that need to be done. Coupled with this, the radiologists have the added pressure of reporting all those scans so that the appropriate management can be made. Hence, if you go in hammer and tongs, you might not be very successful.

It is also worth noting that the radiologist may not necessarily communicate your conversation to the radiographer. It is therefore vital that you write down your reasons for the request (i.e. the patient history and examination findings) and the reasons for the scan (i.e. the differential you are considering). This will help the radiographer to better tailor the scan to that patient.

Fraz, FY1 *"Get good at requesting scans and getting them authorised. Radiology love asking questions; you need to be asking for an appropriate scan for an appropriate history. There is no point talking about a patient with right iliac fossa pain and asking for a CT brain. They will raise those issues, so be precise about the clinical indication and radiology will be more than amenable. There are limited resources and limited slots, if you advocate for your patient, they know you are not just requesting willy-nilly – it's all about having the right approach with people."*

SBAR

These tips for negotiating can be applied when discussing patients with any colleague from a different speciality – and this is a daily occurrence. In this respect, the SBAR (Situation, Background, Assessment, Recommendation) approach is recommended (Crocker et al. 2010).

- **Situation** – your name, grade, calling about (patient and their location), *"the reason for call is . . . "*
- **Background** – include when the patient was admitted and relevant history and background, e.g. medications, blood results, tests or surgical procedures.
- **Assessment** – what you found on examination, e.g. MEWS 4, what has changed and your interpretation.
- **Recommendation** – what you think the patient may need, or what you need advice on. An action plan should then be agreed.

The aim of SBAR is to make communication more succinct. It is particularly useful in high-risk situations (see Box 6.1). This is something you can practise on the wards with a fellow student. Akin to summarising findings, SBAR is something you will require on a daily basis.

Box 6.1

SBAR Example: Dr Coe is an FY1 working on a surgical ward. He calls his registrar about a patient who has developed an irregular heart rhythm.

S: Hi my name is Dr Coe, I am an FY1 calling about Mr Brown on Ward 33, bed 2. I'm concerned about a fast, irregular heart rhythm he has developed.

B: Mr Brown is a 54-year-old gentleman admitted 4 days ago for a total hip replacement. His surgery was successful and there were no post-op complications. He is on 100 mg of Atenolol for hypertension.

A: His heart rate is irregular, his blood pressure is 140/80, he had some shortness of breath and desaturated to 88% on air, but I have stabilised him on 2 L of oxygen. He denies any chest pain or calf pain. The ECG shows atrial fibrillation with a rate of 126 bpm. I am worried he might have a pulmonary embolus.

R: I have ordered a chest Xray and sent off routine bloods to rule out infection and included clotting. Do you think he needs a CTPA? I need your advice on how to proceed.

Professional conflicts

Clare, Consultant *"Conflicts happen all the time: either due to conflicts of interest or difficulties because of personalities. As long as you remain professional and don't personalise any issues, addressing problems objectively, you should be able to resolve them. If you are unable to resolve a problem, then raise it to the appropriate senior. Work is a completely professional place. You don't have to be friends with everyone at work, but you can be friendly at work."*

If you have a concern about a colleague but are unsure how to raise it you can consider the following options (GMC 2008c):
1. Ask a senior or impartial colleague, e.g. your educational supervisor or consultant, for advice.
2. Contact your medical defence body or professional association such as the BMA.
3. Contact the GMC for confidential advice.
4. Contact Public Concern at Work: a charity which provides free, confidential legal advice.

Craig, FY2 *"We were working as a team of four – one colleague was worried about practical stuff and the other was very confident and they really clashed. She felt he didn't pick up his fair load of work, and he felt she wasn't any good. They ended up having a slanging match in front of the patients and the SHO – who rightly told them off. Over the next 2–3 days, the four of us had to work out how we were going to work together. In the end they never really got on but we came up with a way of dividing up the jobs evenly so we all knew what we had to do. We would lend a hand if we finished early,*

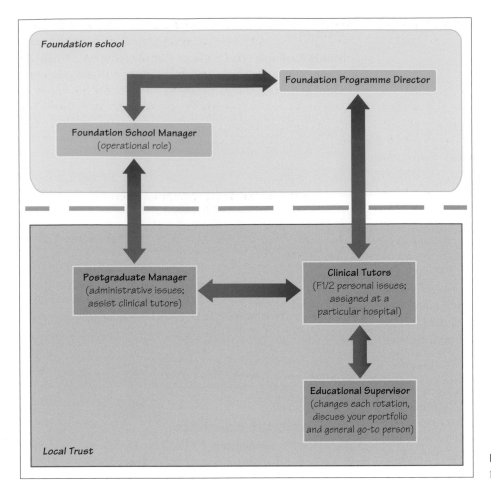

Figure 6.2 The generic structure of a foundation school

but they never helped one another out. It's not an ideal situation, but we found a practical way for them to work side by side. We did our best to resolve the problem amongst ourselves, and I don't think it went any higher than our immediate seniors, so I don't think the consultants or registrars knew about it. If you can try and sort it out at a lower level, then do. If that doesn't work, then raise it at a higher level with your educational supervisor or consultant – but you have to be really sure that there is a need for it because stuff like that does tend to stick. They will remember it and pass judgement. At the end of the day, we are all adults and should be able to sort things amongst ourselves most of the time."

Seeking support

Matthew, Educational Supervisor *"If you feel you are struggling, every deanery should have a 'doctors in difficulty' programme. The unit is well financed for those who need it. If you realise you are struggling it is better to get help earlier rather than later. You don't want to make a mistake and get referred in via another mechanism."*

It is fundamental that you seek help from your seniors on the wards. Likewise, there are external team members who are always there to help you out.

The foundation school

There is a whole network of professionals within every foundation school to facilitate your training and your personal and professional development. Although the number of professionals varies with each school, Figure 6.2 gives you a rough idea of the school's structure. This will aid your understanding of the different roles for the SJT – without overcomplicating matters.

If you have any issue as a foundation doctor, it is always best to go through your educational supervisor or clinical tutor. Liaising between managers is best done internally.

The Foundation Programme Director is the head of the foundation school and ensures that:
• National (UKFPO) and deanery (e.g. Northern) policy are applied to the foundation school.
• The training programme covers the curriculum.
• The foundation school curriculum is delivered to trainees.
• Educational supervisors are up to the proper standards.
• The quality of all aspects of the foundation programme from the configuration of rotations to the spread of specialties available for training is assured.
With respect to your direct needs, your educational supervisor is typically first port of call with:
• Career advice.
• Issues of stress and workload.

- Interpersonal problems, e.g. pregnancy, family difficulties, financial difficulties.
- Lack of training.
- Completing eportfolios.
- Conflicts within your team, e.g. difficult registrar, a lazy FY1.

Most issues can be dealt with by your educational supervisor. If not then your educational supervisor the supervisor may decide to escalate further to the clinical tutors and then to the foundation programme director. Although this is the typical procedure, you can always approach your clinical tutors or foundation programme director directly if you wish. They do have a wider realm of responsibility though, so it is probably best to seek advice from your educational supervisor as they will be able to help you in the most time-efficient manner.

Dan, Foundation Programme Director "*Most major issues get filtered up to me. For example we had one GP practice where the trainees were having a particularly hard time – to the point that they were being bullied by one practitioner. This was sorted locally by the clinical tutors and we no longer send doctors there, but I was still aware of it. There aren't many circumstances in which you would need to contact me directly. If I do receive things, I usually forward them to the relevant clinical tutor as they are on site to deal with the issue. Often I am away visiting other foundation schools or in meetings etc. If you can't get hold of your educational supervisor in the first instance – or they are the problem – your clinical tutors are who you should be contacting.*"

TOP 5 TIPS ON TEAMWORK:

1. Understand your role as part of a team.
2. Facilitate teamwork with good communication between the team players.
3. Help out your colleagues – it's about give and take.
4. Try to sort out conflicts amongst yourselves before you escalate.
5. Your educational supervisor is your first port of call for support.

How do I approach the SJT questions?

Having read this book you should have valuable insight into the types of scenarios you will be asked about, what is expected of you as a FY1, and the knowledge with which to evaluate any question. Although it is important to establish a method that best works for you, the following structure is one of the ways you may wish to approach the SJT:

1. Is this a "ranking" or a "selecting" question? It is important that you answer correctly!

2. Which options are the least appropriate? This will minimise your options and aid your decision.

3. What is expected of me at this level? For example, you are not expected to break bad news as a FY1.

4. Of the options remaining – decide which option is first by thinking: "*if I can only do one thing . . . which would be the most important action to take?*"

5. Then cover this answer up and think: "*If I can no longer do that one, what is now the most important action to take that will resolve this situation?*" and so on. "Should" and "most appropriate" imply ranking in order of importance rather than how you "would" go about tackling the situation in practice. For instance, on the wards it may be that you would speak to a nurse first for advice about a difficult patient as they are often the nearest to hand. In the scenarios, however, you should approach a more senior member of the team first such as a registrar or consultant, as they are more likely to be appropriately equipped to deal with a particular situation.

This question tests your knowledge of transfusion protocol. On the basis of the reasoning set out earlier in this chapter:

1. This is a ranking question.

2. It is not appropriate for someone else to fill in the patient's details as this could potentially cause serious harm if the wrong patient were identified. This would be irresponsible and put the patient at risk. 'A' is therefore last.

3. B is also definitely not appropriate as although you could perhaps identify the sample with your handwriting, this is not something you should do as this could again put the patient at risk.

4. D is the most appropriate option and would immediately resolve the problem. This option will ensure patient safety and leave fewer margins for error. You will know yourself which patient is the right patient and can correctly fill in the form at the bedside.

5. E is the next most appropriate option. This is a perfect opportunity to teach medical students about the mistakes that can happen and the consequences of error in blood transfusion. Ideally, however, you should take the student to the patient rather than sending them with the details. You know the patient – this will ensure that they are correctly identified.

6. This leaves 'C' in the middle. Medicine is about teamwork and it is important to know when it is appropriate to delegate tasks. However, the nurses will also be busy and bloods are primarily an FY1's responsibility, hence this is less appropriate than D and E.

7. The answer is therefore **DECBA**.

SJT example questions

1. An 8-year-old boy comes into A&E with a badly broken leg. He needs surgery. You speak to his parents about the surgery. They explain that they are Jehovah's Witnesses and they don't want their son to have a blood transfusion. What *should* you do?

Rank the following responses from most appropriate (=1) to least appropriate (=5):

A. Inform your consultant about the situation

B. Consult local hospital guidelines on bloodless procedures

C. Ignore the parents' wishes and treat the child in his best interests

D. Tell the parents that it is unlikely that their son will need a transfusion and they should agree to surgery

E. Tell the parents you will see what you can do

---

2. You are working in a haematology clinic. You have been seeing Mrs Alcock regularly over the past 3 months. She says she would like to express her gratitude and hands you a £50 cheque. What *should* you do?

Here is an example:

You are on call in A&E. You have been very busy and failed to fully complete the patient's hospital ID number on the blood bank request form. The lab rings to ask you to rectify the error. The patient requires a "cross-match" because they are due for surgery. What **should** you do?

Rank these responses in order from most appropriate to least appropriate:

A. Apologise and ask the laboratory staff to kindly fill in the patient ID for you.

B. Go to the lab to complete the details yourself.

C. Ask a competent nurse to rebleed the patient as you are busy.

D. Rebleed the patient yourself and rewrite the blood form for cross-match.

E. Send a medical student with the patient details to practice their venepuncture and to report back to you with the bloods.

The Situational Judgement Test at a Glance, First Edition. Frances Varian and Lara Cartwright.

56 © 2013 John Wiley & Sons, Ltd. Published 2013 by John Wiley & Sons, Ltd.

Rank the following responses from most appropriate (=1) to least appropriate (=5):

A. Accept the gift with thanks

B. Politely decline the gift as it is too much

C. Put the money towards a staff night out for everyone to enjoy

D. Say it is hospital policy not to accept monetary gifts

E. Record in the notes you accepted a monetary gift

---

3. You are taking blood from a 70-year-old woman on the medical ward who was admitted following a fall. While you are making conversation about her home circumstances, she tells you that she recently moved in with her son after her husband died. You enquire into how she is coping, and she becomes tearful, telling you that her son has started drinking and becomes very violent when intoxicated. This is the first time she has been in hospital for injuries caused by her son. Her son has assured her he will stop drinking so she doesn't want to make a fuss. What *should* you do?

Rank the following responses from most appropriate (=1) to least appropriate (=5):

A. Inform the nurse in charge about the situation

B. Find out whether she has anyone else she could stay with

C. Contact your specialty trainee (registrar)

D. Give her contact details of a local domestic support group

E. Record details of your conversation in the notes

---

4. A 14-year-old girl attends the GUM clinic asking for an STI check. Before you take some swabs, she tells you that she is pregnant. You confirm this with a pregnancy test. You ask her whether she has told anyone; she says no and that she especially doesn't want her parents to know. What *should* you do?

Rank the following responses from most appropriate (=1) to least appropriate (=5):

A. Tell her that you have to let her parents know because she is under sixteen

B. Try to persuade her it would be in her best interests to tell her parents

C. Tell her that you will respect her wishes and not tell anyone

D. Ask your consultant to see her

E. Advise her that you are obliged to let her GP know

---

5. The family of one of your patients who died is registering a complaint about their treatment. The solicitor calls you and asks for the medical records of the deceased to be sent to him. What *should* you do?

Rank the following responses from most appropriate (=1) to least appropriate (=5):

A. Send over the records as requested

B. Say that you will get someone senior to call them back and take their details

C. Remind them that any requests need to be sent in writing to the legal department

D. Call your consultant and ask them to speak to the solicitor

E. Take the solicitor's details and tell them you will get the nurse to fax over the information

---

6. You are in outpatients and you realise that your mobile phone has been stolen. You suspect one of eight patients could have taken it. You ring your insurance company and they tell you that you need to call the police and get a crime reference number. You call them, but cannot get a number without giving the police the names of the individuals in outpatients that day. What *should* you do?

Rank the following responses from most appropriate (=1) to least appropriate (=5):

A. Give over the names of the patients so that you can make a claim

B. Fill in a critical incident (CAE) form

C. Accuse patients you suspect and question them about it

D. Ignore it and just replace your phone

E. Report the incident to the foundation director

---

7. A 16-year-old girl comes into A&E with diabetic ketoacidosis (DKA). She is admitted and treated. The following morning you are arranging her discharge. You discuss her diabetic control with her. She says that she can't be bothered with the insulin as it's too much hassle. What *should* you do?

Rank the following responses from most appropriate (=1) to least appropriate (=5):

A. Educate her about the importance of compliance

B. Arrange for the specialist diabetic nurse to see her before she goes

C. Make a note of her non-compliance on the discharge summary to the GP

D. Ask her parents to speak to her about compliance if they come to collect her

E. Ask her why the insulin is such a problem

---

8. A 32-year-old woman presents to A&E for a head laceration. She claims that her boyfriend hit her, and she fell and hit her head. You smell alcohol on her breath. On questioning you find that she has left her two children at home under the supervision of her boyfriend who has also been drinking. You are worried about the children, what *should* you do?

Rank the following responses from most appropriate (=1) to least appropriate (=5):

A. Call social services to report your concern

B. Call your registrar to assess the mother and discuss the case

C. Fill in a referral form for social services

D. Tell the mother it is protocol that you put in a referral to social services

E. Tell the mother that you are concerned about the children, given her injuries

9. Mrs Smith is 53-year-old lady who suffered with heart failure for many years. She has expressed a wish to receive no further treatment and go home to rest in peace. The nurse comes to see you the following day, saying that her husband has arrived and is angry that you are sending her home to die. He feels his wife is "out of her mind and not thinking straight". What *should* you do?

Rank the following responses from most appropriate (=1) to least appropriate (=5):

A. Go and see Mrs Smith to find out whether she remains firm in her wishes

B. Ask the nurse to inform the husband it is Mrs Smith's decision

C. Explore the husband's concerns

D. Refer to psychiatry

E. Persuade Mrs Smith to go with you to speak to her husband about her wishes

10. Your FY1 colleague Mark has turned up late again for handover, and you smell alcohol on his breath. You know he has been having some family problems recently. You suspect the alcohol is from last night, but you cannot be sure. What *should* you do?

Rank the following responses from most appropriate (=1) to least appropriate (=5):

A. Report Mark immediately to the foundation programme director

B. Ask your educational supervisor for advice

C. Suggest to Mark that he explain the situation to the specialty trainee (registrar)

D. Report the situation immediately to your consultant

E. Have a quiet word with Mark after the handover to ask how he is coping

11. An elderly woman is brought in by ambulance to A&E. She doesn't speak English. The paramedics say that she was found collapsed on the street and a passer-by called 999. She is stable, but you suspect she needs to be kept in overnight. You name some languages and she nods at "Urdu". It is 7.30 p.m., what *should* you do?

Rank the following responses from most appropriate (=1) to least appropriate (=5):

A. Arrange for an interpreter to come to the hospital

B. Use an online translation service

C. See if the patient can contact a friend or relative to interpret

D. Arrange for a telephone interpretation

E. Find a colleague on the ward and see if they can translate

12. You are working on an oncology ward. It is a Saturday night and a patient is asking you for the results of his myeloma screen. The nurse tells you that the patient is going to complain if they do not get the results soon. The patient is anxious and cannot understand why it is taking so long. You do not have their results yet. What *should* you do?

Rank the following responses from most appropriate (=1) to least appropriate (=5):

A. Explain to the patient it is unlikely you will get the results before Monday

B. Tell the nurse to go and explain to the patient that it is not possible to get the results until Monday

C. Call the laboratory and put an urgent on the results

D. Call the registrar and ask them to speak to the patient

E. Apologise to the patient for the delay but explain that it is a weekend and unfortunately you will not have the results until Monday

13. You are working on a respiratory ward. A locum consultant prescribes antibiotics for Mr Jones for community-acquired pneumonia. You know these particular antibiotics are outside hospital guidelines. What *should* you do?

Rank the following responses from most appropriate (=1) to least appropriate (=5):

A. Prescribe the treatment as the consultant wishes but document in the notes they are outside of hospital guidelines

B. Show the guidelines to the consultant and ask whether the antibiotics should still be prescribed

C. Ask the consultant the reasons for prescribing those antibiotics

D. Follow the guidelines and ignore the consultant's prescription

E. Ring pharmacy and find out their recommendations

14. You are working a night shift on a surgical ward. A patient already on treatment for sepsis starts to rapidly deteriorate. It is nearly midnight. You complete your A to E primary survey and the patient is stable for the moment, but you feel you are out of your depth. You call the surgical registrar, but they tell you to call the medical team because they are busy in theatre. When you bleep the on-call medical registrar, they tell you it is not their responsibility and to find someone else. What *should* you do?

Rank the following responses from most appropriate (=1) to least appropriate (=5):

A. Call the surgical consultant at home

B. Start basic management for the patient

C. Call the surgical registrar again, explain the situation and ask for advice

D. Ask a nurse to arrange for someone to help you

E. Put out a periarrest call on 2222

15. A patient with end-stage motor neurone disease asks you to give them the lethal injection. You explain to them that this is not legal in this country. What *should* you do?

Rank the following responses from most appropriate (=1) to least appropriate (=5):

A. Explore the patient's reasons for wanting the lethal injection

B. Tell the patient's partner how they feel

C. Ask the patient to talk to their partner about their feelings

D. Refer the patient to psychiatry

E. Explain to the patient about an advance directive and start the process

---

16. An 83-year-old man is brought in to A&E after a fall. He has severe dementia and is obviously in pain, but is unable to tell you where the pain is coming from. After examination you suspect he has a broken hip. This is confirmed by X-ray. A decision needs to be made about treatment. However, he lacks capacity. His wife is deceased and his daughter, detailed as his next of kin, lives in Australia. What *should* you do?

Rank the following responses from most appropriate (=1) to least appropriate (=5):

A. Contact your local Independent Mental Capacity Advocate (IMCA) organisation

B. Try to contact his daughter in Australia

C. Speak to the registrar about scheduling him onto the surgical list

D. Check through the notes for any legal documentation

E. Start treatment anyway and give him analgesia

---

17. It is a quiet afternoon on your surgical ward. The consultant asks you to come and assist with a private list in the afternoon at a different hospital. What *should* you do?

Rank the following responses from most appropriate (=1) to least appropriate (=5):

A. Ask your educational supervisor for advice

B. Agree to help your consultant

C. Decline and go down to the theatres to see if you can assist with any surgical cases

D. Decline because you have responsibilities on the ward

E. Ask your fellow FY1 colleague for advice

---

18. You are seeing a patient in minors in A&E on a Friday night. A nurse comes in to tell you that a patient is being verbally aggressive and threatening because they haven't been seen yet and thinks people are "jumping the queue". The nurse suspects the patient has been drinking alcohol. What *should* you do?

Rank the following responses from most appropriate (=1) to least appropriate (=5):

A. Go and see the patient and tell them they will not be treated unless they calm down

B. Ask the nurse to call security

C. Tell the nurse to get someone else to see the patient because you are too busy

D. Explain to the patient that you are very busy but that you will see them as soon as possible

E. Physically restrain the patient

---

19. A 60-year-old Indian man comes into A&E with a history of fits. He was discharged 2 days ago from ITU. His wife is with him, but she does not speak English. He is very confused, disorientated and, from your A to E assessment, clearly unwell. You cannot get a history. It is 4 p.m. on a Monday afternoon. What *should* you do?

Rank the following responses from most appropriate (=1) to least appropriate (=5):

A. Proceed anyway with routine examination and investigations

B. Ring the GP to get background information on the patient

C. Ring the patient's family to obtain the information

D. Ask ITU to fax over their notes from the previous admission

E. Arrange for an interpreter before you proceed

---

20. You are working as an FY1 on an obstetrics and gynaecology ward. A 29-year-old woman is admitted four hours into labour. This is her first pregnancy. She is requesting a Caesarean section (CS), but there is no medical indication for it at this stage. This is different from her birth plan, but the patient is demanding that she be given the care that she wants. What *should* you do?

Rank these responses from most appropriate to (=1) to least appropriate (=5):

A. Ask a midwife on the ward for advice

B. Ring the consultant obstetrician to make them aware of the situation

C. Explore the patient's reasons for wanting a CS

D. Explain the overall risks and benefits of both a CS and vaginal birth

E. Refuse the CS as it is not medically indicated

---

21. A 27-year-old woman comes into A&E with vomiting and mild abdominal pain. You have sent off bloods, but in the meantime the routine pregnancy test comes back positive. Her fiancé rings casualty to ask how she is doing. What *should* you do?

Rank the following responses from most appropriate (=1) to least appropriate (=5):

A. Tell her partner that she is pregnant

B. Tell her partner that it is nothing serious and that she will be fine

C. Tell her partner that he will have to speak to his fiancée directly

D. Tell her partner that you will need to get her consent before you tell him anything

E. Tell her partner that you are still waiting for the results of all the investigations

22. You are an FY1 working on the gastroenterology ward. A nurse comes to tell you that one of the patients with chronic alcoholism has been very rude. This is not the first time it has happened. The nurse is clearly quite upset, what *should* you do?

Rank the following responses from most appropriate (=1) to least appropriate (=5):

A. Tell the nurse you will speak to the patient

B. Go and speak to the patient and tell them their behaviour is unacceptable

C. Advise the nurse to ignore it

D. Advise the nurse to avoid them and work in a different section

E. Ask the patient to apologise to the nurse

---

23. A patient – well known to psychiatry – is admitted onto the gastro ward with a history of somatisation disorder (multiple physical complaints with a psychological cause). She is demanding a bowel resection following a colonoscopy. The results of the colonoscopy are completely normal, and surgery is not clinically indicated. She is angry that you will not treat her and threatens to "cut it out herself if you don't". What *should* you do?

Rank the following responses from most appropriate (=1) to least appropriate (=5):

A. Agree with the patient that if she calms down you will consider surgery

B. Bleep the on-call psychiatrist

C. Reiterate to the patient that you cannot operate because the colonoscopy was normal

D. Explain to the patient that, given the normal tests, you think this is part of their mental health problem

E. Call the senior registrar for advice

---

24. You are working as an FY1 in a GUM clinic. You are seeing a young man with newly diagnosed Hepatitis B. He is an ex-intravenous drug user who works in a bar. You question him about his partner and discover that he has not disclosed his Hepatitis B status as he is afraid this will mean his partner will leave him. He says they are having protected sexual intercourse. What *should* you do?

Rank the following responses from most appropriate (=1) to least appropriate (=5):

A. Try to persuade him to tell his partner

B. Do not disclose any information as there is no risk to his partner

C. Explain you have a duty to tell his partner about their risk of infection

D. Offer to talk to the patient and his partner together

E. Recommend counselling

---

25. You are an FY1 working on a labour ward. One of your patients has a breech presentation. She has a birth plan which specifies that every appropriate method should be attempted before opting for a Caesarean section (CS). She has now changed her mind and decided to have a CS. Her husband disagrees; taking you to one side and saying "she's in pain, she doesn't know what she wants, she'll regret it if you operate". What *should* you do?

Rank the following responses from most appropriate (=1) to least appropriate (=5):

A. Inform her of the overall risks and benefits of a CS and vaginal birth

B. Call the consultant obstetrician to review the patient

C. Enquire into her reasons for the change in birth plan

D. Tell the husband you accept his point and remind him that it is his wife's choice not his

E. Ask the husband to leave so that you can speak to your patient in private

---

26. You are working on a gastroenterology ward and a nurse approaches you and says Mr Brown needs to be prescribed his usual fluids. You are finishing up a discharge summary and take home drugs for another patient. What *should* you do?

Rank the following responses from most appropriate (=1) to least appropriate (=5):

A. Prescribe Mr Brown normal saline

B. Go and see Mr Brown straight away

C. Explain that, to enable you to get the discharges done on time, they should ask another FY1 to help

D. Say you will put it on your jobs list and get to it as soon as you can

E. Ask about Mr Brown's fluid status

---

27. A colleague has left 30 minutes early to attend a dental appointment. They have asked you to prescribe Warfarin for their patient. Your shift has already ended, and you were about to go home. The INR result from the morning's blood tests is not back yet. What *should* you do?

Rank the following responses from most appropriate (=1) to least appropriate (=5):

A. Prescribe the Warfarin anyway

B. Hand over the request to the ward cover

C. Write it onto your jobs list for the morning

D. Write that the patient needs their Warfarin dosing in their notes

E. Ring the lab to see if the INR results are there

---

28. You are working as an FY1 on a surgical ward. On your way to ordering a CT scan from radiology, you are bleeped. You find the nearest phone to ring through. A nurse is concerned about Mrs Fazi's urine output (UO). You remember it was fine for her small frame when you checked two hours ago. What *should* you do?

Rank the following responses from most appropriate (=1) to least appropriate (=5):

A. Ask the nurse to do some basic observations on Mrs Fazi and say you will come as soon as you have ordered the CT scan

B. Go and see Mrs Fazi straight away

C. Reassure the nurse that Mrs Fazi's UO was fine for her size two hours ago

D. Ask the nurse whether Mrs Fazi's UO has changed since this morning

E. Tell the nurse to start 1 litre of normal saline over 8 hours for Mrs Fazi, and you will prescribe it once you have been to radiology

---

29. You go to see a patient with whom you previously had trouble putting in a cannula. You ask them whether you can take some blood. They recognise you and say "don't come anywhere near me with that thing, you don't know what you're doing". What *should* you do?

Rank the following responses from most appropriate (=1) to least appropriate (=5):

A. Reassure the patient that you are competent at taking blood

B. Go and ask a nurse to take their blood

C. Apologise to the patient for yesterday

D. Tell the patient you have to take their blood as there is no one else

E. Take the blood from their cannula

---

30. A patient you recently discharged from the ward requests your friendship on a social networking site. They are a similar age to you. What *should* you do?

Rank the following responses from most appropriate (=1) to least appropriate (=5):

A. Accept the friend request but do not engage with the former patient

B. Decline the friend request and explain your reasons

C. Ignore their friend request

D. Ask your FY1 colleagues for advice

E. Ask your educational supervisor for advice

---

31. You are working on ITU, completing the morning's job list. When taking bloods from a patient – admitted following a road traffic accident – you accidently stick yourself with the needle. You had followed infection control guidelines and were wearing gloves, but you see your finger bleeding underneath. You quickly squeeze it, clean it and put a dressing on it. You go to look on the system for anything on the patient's HIV/Hepatitis status but there is nothing. The patient is unconscious. What *should* you do?

Choose the **three** most appropriate options from the following list:

A. Request viral serology on the blood forms for HIV and Hepatitis status

B. Ring occupational health

C. Go down to A&E to get some anti-retrovirals to start immediately

D. Fill in a CAE form for the stick injury

E. Ask if you can go home because you are so worried

F. Wait to see if the patient wakes up and ask their permission for serology

G. Bleep your registrar to explain the situation

H. Explain to one of the nurses what has happened

---

32. Your FY1 colleague turns up late again for their shift. The ward you are working on is quiet. Your colleague arrives in tears; she is feeling exhausted, stressed and says that she is not coping with anything at the minute. This is the third time in the past two weeks. What *should* you do?

Choose the **three** most appropriate options from the following list:

A. Apologise and say that you are busy now but that you will talk to her after your shift

B. Sit her down to have a talk about her problems

C. Suggest she books an appointment to see her GP

D. Suggest she speaks to her registrar

E. Suggest she takes sick leave

F. Advise her to talk to her educational supervisor

G. Seek advice about the situation from your educational supervisor

H. Mention that you have to inform your consultant of her difficulties

---

33. You are working in Children's A&E on a Saturday night. A 13-year-old boy comes in drunk. He admits he has been drinking alcohol and says he fell over. The X-ray confirms he has broken his index and middle fingers. The boy is adamant he is fine and doesn't want any treatment because he is scared that his parents will find out he has been drinking. He wants you to just give him some pain-killers and then he'll leave. What *should* you do?

Choose the top **three** most appropriate options from the following list:

A. Prescribe the painkillers and let him self-discharge

B. Ring the boy's parents without telling him

C. Explain that you really need to let his parents know what has happened and it would be best if he rang them

D. Tell him to go and see his GP if he has any problems over the weekend

E. Try to persuade him to have his fingers splinted

F. Put in a referral for social services

G. Refuse to let him self-discharge without getting the proper treatment

H. Discuss the situation with the nurse in charge

34. You are on a ward round with your consultant on the coronary care unit. The patient's relatives are sitting in the waiting room at the end of the corridor. Your consultant says that the patient is going to die soon and checks the Do Not Attempt Resuscitation (DNAR) form. The family approach you politely after the ward round whilst you are ordering bloods and say "so you think Mum is going to die, do you?" It is clear they have overheard your consultant's comments. What *should* you do?

Choose the **three** most appropriate options from the following list:

A. Ask a nurse to take the family to a side room and explain you will follow shortly

B. Ask them where they heard that information

C. Tell them you are busy at the moment and will talk to them later

D. Apologise to the family for the fact that they overheard the conversation with your consultant

E. Fill in a critical incident (CAE) form

F. Ask the family if they would like to sit with their mum

G. Finish ordering the bloods

H. Call your consultant, explain what happened and ask them to speak to the family

35. A 9-year-old boy was admitted following an exacerbation of asthma. You speak with the parents about using his steroid inhaler. The boy's mother is happy to make sure he has the inhaler; however, his father is clearly not. Father says that he has heard that they will stunt his boy's growth and he doesn't want that. What *should* you do?

Choose the **three** most appropriate options from the following list:

A. Ignore the father's wishes and prescribe the inhaler anyway as the mother has consented

B. Contact social services about the disagreement

C. Ask the asthma specialist nurse for advice

D. Agree with the father not to use the steroid inhaler

E. Get the mother to persuade the father the steroid inhaler is necessary

F. Plan to monitor the boy's growth on a growth chart and review throughout the use of his inhaler

G. Educate the father about the advantages to using the inhaler

H. Ask the boy what he would like to do

36. A 43-year-old man is brought in by ambulance to A&E after collapsing in a bar on a Friday night. You have no details other than his name and date of birth, which the paramedics got from his wallet. The man is incapable of giving a history due to his level of intoxication. He is stable in the resuscitation area. What *should* you do?

Choose the **three** most appropriate options from the following list:

A. Continue with your A to E assessment

B. Ring your specialty registrar

C. Ask a clerk to search the hospital database for his records

D. Search through his mobile phone contacts to find a family number and call them

E. Start treatment anyway

F. Call the cardiac on-call SHO

G. Start the appropriate investigations but do not start any new medications

H. Ask one of the nurses to try and track down some information on him

37. A 24-year-old woman is admitted to A&E following a paracetamol overdose. Her boyfriend brought her in when she admitted that she had taken 50×500 mg paracetamol tablets one hour earlier. Her boyfriend tells you she has been suffering from depression. You speak with her alone and she refuses any form of treatment – she wants to die. What *should* you do?

Choose the **three** most appropriate options from the following list:

A. Respect her right to refuse treatment

B. See if her boyfriend can persuade her to change her mind

C. Bleep the on-call psychiatrist

D. Call your registrar

E. Treat her under the Mental Health Act

F. Treat her under the Mental Capacity Act

G. Treat her under the doctrine of necessity

H. Discharge her from A&E

38. You are working on a labour ward as an FY1. A nurse comes to see you to let you know that the ex-partner of one of the mothers is demanding to see his baby in the special care baby unit. He wasn't present at the birth, and you know that the mother hasn't been in contact with him since she became pregnant. What *should* you do?

Choose the **three** most appropriate options for the following list:

A. Take him to see the baby because he is the father

B. Check the baby's birth certificate and ask to see some identification to confirm who he is

C. Ask the mother to confirm whether he is the father

D. Ask the midwife what you should do

E. Ring the registrar and ask for advice

F. Document in the notes that this man wanted access to the child

G. Tell the man that he will have to come back another time once he has pre-arranged a visit

H. Tell the man that he cannot see the baby until you have spoken to the mother

39. A 79-year-old male is awaiting surgical repair of a fractured neck of femur. He tells you that he is a Jehovah's Witness and says he will refuse the operation if he needs a blood transfusion. **You suspect the risk of needing a blood transfusion is high. He asks if there are any other options. What *should* you do?**

Choose the **three** most appropriate options from the following list:

A. Explain the consequences to him of not having the operation

B. Ask his permission to contact the local Hospital Liaison Committee (HLC)

C. Advise him to contact the Watchtower Society for information

D. Tell him that you are unsure of the options but that you will find out

E. Take bloods and order routine pre-op investigations

F. Bleep your registrar to review the patient

G. Consult your local policy guidance on bloodless medical procedures

H. Find out why he is opposed to a blood transfusion and what his preferences are on the use of blood products

---

40. **A man is sitting in minors in A&E after having a drunken brawl with his friend. He has superficial lacerations to his shoulder and forearm. He arrived at midnight and, having been waiting for three hours, is getting increasingly agitated. The nurse comes to tell you that he is angry and threatening to self-discharge. You are busy packing the nose of his friend whom he was fighting with. What *should* you do?**

Choose the **three** most appropriate options from the following list:

A. Allow him to self-discharge, you do not respond to threats

B. Ask the nurse to let the patient know that he is next

C. Call security

D. Apologise to him for the long wait and thank him for his patience

E. Tell the nurse to get the suture kit ready

F. Ask the nurse to tell him he should wait because you are seeing to his friend

G. Leave his friend and go and attend to his shoulder and forearm lacerations

H. Call the SHO to review and suture him

---

41. **You are in the surgical assessment unit, trying to consent a 55-year-old man for rigid sigmoidoscopy that you will be doing under supervision. You have been trained to consent for this procedure and are aware of all the risks and benefits. When you try to explain the procedure, he says "do whatever you think is best, Doc, I don't want to know". What *should* you do?**

Choose the **three** most appropriate options from the following list:

A. Tell him you need to give him a brief explanation of the procedure

B. Ask him to sign the form without going into detail

C. Tell him it is important that he understands the procedure in order to consent

D. Phone your registrar to consent the patient

E. Ask him whether he would prefer a family member with him whilst you explain the procedure

F. Explain the procedure to a family member instead

G. Cancel the investigation as you cannot go ahead without consent

H. Fill in the form yourself and sign it in his best interests

---

42. **You are looking after Mrs Chang, who is intermittently confused. Her family are all in the waiting room and are anxious to know how she is doing. You have the results of her CT scan which is normal. What *should* you do?**

Choose the **three** most appropriate options from the following list:

A. Go and tell Mrs Chang's family the good news

B. Go see Mrs Chang to find out how she is today

C. Ask a nurse to go and tell the family the good news

D. Tell Mrs Chang's family how she is generally doing, but say that you cannot give them any specific results until you have spoken to Mrs Chang

E. Wait until Mrs Chang's family ask specifically about her results

F. Let your colleagues know Mrs Chang's results

G. View the scan yourself

H. Ring the registrar to ask for advice

---

43. **You are working on an oncology ward. You are sitting at the desk ordering bloods when your colleague Jane tells you she thinks that you are not picking up your fair share of work. You feel Jane is boisterous and arrogant. No one else has mentioned anything to you about being lazy, and you feel you are competent. What *should* you do?**

Choose the **three** most appropriate options from the following list:

A. Be honest with Jane that you think she is arrogant

B. Argue with Jane that you do your fair share

C. Say you cannot discuss this here and suggest a more appropriate place

D. Suggest that you divide the jobs evenly

E. Ask Jane why she feels you are not doing your share

F. Raise the issue with your educational supervisor

G. Ask your other colleagues their opinion of you

H. Report the bullying to your consultant

---

44. **You are working on a busy respiratory ward. One of your colleagues, Jack, is consistently lazy to the point where he may be compromising patient care. The nurses and ward cover at handover have commented on this. What *should* you do?**

Choose the **three** most appropriate options from the following list:

A. Offer to take on some of Jack's workload

B. Ask Jack whether he feels he is struggling

C. Tell Jack he is not doing his share of the workload

D. Inform the foundation programme clinical lead

E. Recommend the nurse in charge has a quiet word

F. Ask the nurses to fill in a Clinically Adverse Event (CAE) form

G. Inform your consultant that Jack is struggling

H. Tell Jack you will speak to your educational supervisor if things don't change

---

45. You send a medical student to take some bloods – for which they are trained. You check the results at 3 p.m. and realise that the samples are all coagulated. What *should* you do?

Choose the **three** most appropriate options from the following list:

A. Retake the bloods

B. Report the student to your consultant

C. Point out the mistake to the student when you see them the following day

D. Ignore their mistake

E. Supervise the student when taking blood next time

F. Tell the student to bring the samples to you next time before they send them

G. Suggest the student reflects on this incident in their portfolio

H. Tell the student to get some more clinical skills training before they go on the wards

---

46. You are working in a GP surgery. A patient comes in to see you with symptoms of angina at rest. It says on the system that the GP told them last time not to drive. You ask them whether they have been driving, and they tell you that they have: they drove to the surgery today. What *should* you do?

Choose the **three** most appropriate options from the following list:

A. Report them to the DVLA

B. Advise them to inform the DVLA

C. Advise them to stop driving until their symptoms are under control

D. Find out whether someone can drive them home

E. Ask if they remember the GP advising them not to drive

F. Remind them last time the GP asked them not to drive

G. Speak to the GP for advice

H. Ask them to hand over their keys until someone can drive them home

---

47. Your consultant on a ward round orders a spine MRI and asks you to put in the request. You overhear the registrar saying to another colleague that it is not indicated. What *should* you do?

Choose the **three** most appropriate options from the following list:

A. Order the MRI as the consultant has requested

B. Ask the consultant the reasons for ordering the MRI

C. Ignore the consultant and do as your registrar says

D. Tell the consultant that the registrar does not think the MRI is indicated

E. Ask the registrar why they think the MRI is not indicated

F. Ring the radiologist to discuss the MRI request

G. Ask the registrar to speak to consultant about their difference in opinion

H. Document in the notes that the MRI was ordered but that the registrar disagreed

---

48. You are working as an FY1 as part of the medical on-call team. A patient with type I diabetes came in with diabetic ketoacidosis (DKA), but is improving having been on a sliding-scale. The consultant prescribes short-acting insulin. The patient disagrees with this and asks that he be put back onto his regular insulin regimen of long-acting insulin. What *should* you do?

Choose the **three** most appropriate options from the following list:

A. Ask the specialist diabetic nurse for advice

B. Call the consultant to relay the patient's disapproval of their regimen

C. Prescribe the patient long-acting insulin instead

D. Tell the patient that they are on the right insulin

E. Tell the patient they will have to discuss it with the consultant the next time they see him

F. Write both up on the drug chart to be delivered

G. Ask the patient why they don't want to have short-acting insulin

H. Ignore the patient's request as they are clearly still unwell and confused

---

49. A 69-year-old man is brought into A&E with symptoms later confirmed as an ischaemic stroke. Your specialist registrar reviews him in A&E and writes up his prescription on a drug chart. The patient reaches you on the stroke ward one hour later with his notes and a different drug chart. Clopidogrel is written up STAT but not given. The prescription written is not the one that your registrar wrote. What *should* you do?

Choose the **three** most appropriate options from the following list:

A. Ring pharmacy to ask for advice

B. Bleep your registrar

C. Take the chart down to A&E and look for the other one

D. Ask the patient whether they have been given the Clopidogrel

E. Give the Clopidogrel as it is important they receive urgent anticoagulation

F. Give half the dose of Clopidogrel

G. Delay giving the Clopidogrel until the other chart is found

H. Tell the nurses not to give Clopidogrel to the patient

You are working on a busy cardiology ward. Your colleague is on call and asks you to hold their bleep for them whilst they go and get some lunch. What *should* you do?

Choose the three most appropriate options from the following list?

A. Agree to hold their bleep

B. Offer to go with them for their lunch

C. Politely decline because you have your own patients

D. Suggest they get in touch with someone on the on-call team to hold their bleep

E. See whether they have any outstanding jobs you can help with

F. Offer to get their lunch for them

G. Tell them to turn it off whilst they go and get some lunch

H. Suggest they go quickly to get their lunch

1. An 8-year-old boy comes into A&E with a badly broken leg. He needs surgery. You speak to his parents about the surgery. They explain that they are Jehovah's Witnesses and they don't want their son to have a blood transfusion. What *should* you do?

ANSWER: AEBCD

This question is about respecting and communicating a patient's religious views in such a way as to best accommodate them into clinical care. For more information on Jehovah's Witnesses see Chapter 5. In this scenario you are expected to seek help in a tricky situation.

A. *Informing your consultant* is the most appropriate option as they have to make the final decision in this situation. If you could only choose one of the options in this question, this would be it. Everything else is subsidiary to recognising that you should seek help. The consultant will also be able to advise you on what to tell the parents (E).

E. *Telling the parents you will see what you can do* is the next most appropriate option. It is best practice to value guardians' wishes and respect that they are acting in the best interests of the child – but you should speak to a senior before you say this.

B. *Consulting the local hospital guidelines* is the next most appropriate option as this will further your own learning and development.

C. *Ignoring the parents' wishes* is not appropriate, as they should be respected. Your consultant could override their decision acting in the child's best interests. However, this is an area that would cause considerable conflict and is best avoided.

D. *Telling the parents it is unlikely that their son will need a transfusion* is the least appropriate option. You cannot lie to the parents and you do not know the likelihood of the child needing a transfusion. You also cannot say for definite that this boy won't need one. If the surgery went ahead and he needed blood, then the correct planning would not be in place and you would be going against the parents' (and child's) wishes. This has negative consequences for you as a clinician, and for the patient and their relatives.

---

2. You are working in a haematology clinic. You have been seeing Mrs Alcock regularly over the past 3 months. She says she would like to express her gratitude and hands you a £50 cheque. What *should* you do?

ANSWER: DBECA

The GMC recommends that: "You must not encourage patients to give, lend or bequeath money or gifts that will directly or indirectly benefit you" (GMC 2008a).

D. *Saying it is hospital policy not to accept monetary gifts* is the most appropriate option. Whether or not it is 'officially' hospital policy (in many trusts it is), you should decline the patient's gift in this manner as it shouldn't cause too much offence. If you simply decline the gift because it is too much (B), then the patient might bring £20 next time. Under no circumstances should you accept monetary gifts, as they could be mistaken for a bribe.

B. *Politely declining the gift as 'it is too much'* is the next most appropriate option. £50 is too much money to accept. Although it is nice to receive gifts of gratitude from patients, you should not be accepting large sums of money. Flowers and chocolates as gifts are very different from money: you have to make a sensible judgement on this.

E. *Recording in the notes that you accepted a monetary gift* is the next most appropriate option. Although it is not appropriate to accept such a generous gift, you should record it in the notes if you did, and explain your reasons for accepting the gift.

C. *Putting the money towards a staff night out* is not appropriate. Although, ideally, you should share gifts with your colleagues, you cannot simply accept a monetary donation and record it in another way. Usually patients will bring gifts for the healthcare team, and so this issue is rarely a problem.

A. *Accepting the gift with thanks* is the least appropriate option. This may encourage this patient to give further gifts and things of monetary worth should not be accepted, as this could easily be mistaken as bribery.

---

3. You are taking blood from a 70-year-old woman on the medical ward who was admitted following a fall. While you are making conversation about her home circumstances, she tells you that she recently moved in with her son after her husband died. You enquire into how she is coping, and she becomes tearful, telling you that her son has started drinking and becomes very violent when intoxicated. This is the first time she has been in hospital for injuries caused by her son. Her son has assured her he will stop drinking, so she doesn't want to make a fuss. What *should* you do?

ANSWER: ACEBD

This question is asking you to consider the risk to this elderly lady. An FY1 should always ensure the patient is the focus of care.

A. *Informing the nurse in charge about the situation* is the most appropriate option. This will directly deal with the problem, as the nurses can refer to social services and take the appropriate protective measures for this lady if her son tries to visit her on the ward. Remember that nurses are the guardians of safety and informing them about this lady is the best thing you can do to protect her.

The Situational Judgement Test at a Glance, First Edition. Frances Varian and Lara Cartwright.

66 © 2013 John Wiley & Sons, Ltd. Published 2013 by John Wiley & Sons, Ltd.

C. *Contacting your specialty trainee* is the next most appropriate, as a more senior member of your team can give advice on how to appropriately manage this situation. They should be informed of those situations where patient safety is compromised.

E. *Recording details of your conversation in the notes* is the next most suitable response as you need to record the patient's situation accurately. It is good practice to document everything in the notes including the situation, who you informed and actions taken. This covers you legally, hence the saying: if it's not written down, it never happened!

B. *Finding out whether she has anyone else she can stay with* is the next most appropriate option. Although this finds out more about her social circumstances, it does not formally address the problem. Also, removing her from her current social situation would not be your decision to make. Given her age and fragility, this would require input from social services, OT and physios about the suitability of a move.

D. *Giving her the contact details of a local support group* is not appropriate. There has not been a decision made yet as to how the medical team will best help this lady. Giving her details of a local domestic support group may leave her feeling dismissed as there is much more that can be done to help her. She should not be made to feel as if she has to resolve anything herself at this vulnerable time.

---

4. A 14-year-old girl attends the GUM clinic asking for an STI check. Before you take some swabs, she tells you that she is pregnant. You confirm this with a pregnancy test. You ask her whether she has told anyone; she says no and that she especially doesn't want her parents to know. What *should* you do?

This question is asking you to consider the health of the unborn baby as well as the health of the teenager. Refer to Chapter 2 for more information on under eighteens.

D. *Asking your consultant to see her* is the most appropriate option, as you cannot assess Gillick competence as an FY1. You should recognise that this is a difficult situation and you need senior advice.

B. *Trying to persuade her it would be in her best interests to tell her parents* is the next most appropriate option. Although not every situation will warrant this action – for example, if it was felt telling the parents could potentially harm the teenager – you should have a sensible discussion about this. Ideally she will be able to seek support from her parents.

E. *Advising her that you are obliged to let her GP know* is the next most appropriate option, as you need to consider the health of the unborn baby. This is where the GP steps in. Medical care will be needed throughout the pregnancy, or for any other decisions she may make. Informing her GP may also be a compromise, if she refuses to let her parents know.

C. *Telling her that you will respect her wishes and not tell anyone* is not appropriate. This would be dishonest, given

that you need to at least discuss it with your consultant and the GP.

A. *Telling her that you have to let her parents know because she is under sixteen* is the least appropriate response as you should not break confidentiality without strong justification. If she is Gillick competent, her wish for confidentiality should be respected.

---

5. The family of one of your patients who died is registering a complaint about their treatment. The solicitor calls you and asks for the medical records of the deceased to be sent to him. What *should* you do?

Remember that the duty of confidentiality persists after the patient has died. Moreover, no party has a general right to information, and therefore only information should be provided that is relevant to the claim. No situation where there is a potential breach of confidentiality should ever be rushed. Refer back to Chapter 2 for more information on confidentiality.

C. *Reminding them that any requests need to be sent in writing to the legal department* is the most appropriate option, and the solicitor phoning should be aware of this. This directly – and appropriately – deals with this problem. As an FY1 you should not be involved in the sending of information to third parties, but you can direct them to the appropriate department.

D. *Calling your consultant* is the next most appropriate response, as they can more appropriately deal with this type of request. They would also tell the solicitor to send it in writing to the legal department.

B. *Getting a senior to call them back* is the next most appropriate option. Options include contacting your F1 clinical lead, foundation programme director or foundation programme co-ordinator for legal matters. This action will delay tackling the issue as compared with contacting your consultant.

E. *Faxing over the information* – even if a nurse does it – is not appropriate. It is the legal department's responsibility to deal with this matter, not the medical team's.

A. *Sending over the records as requested* is the least appropriate response as this is a serious breach of confidentiality.

---

6. You are in outpatients and you realise that your mobile phone has been stolen. You suspect one of eight patients could have taken it. You ring your insurance company, and they tell you that you need to call the police and get a crime reference number. You call them but cannot get a number without giving the police the names of the individuals in outpatients that day. What *should* you do?

This question requires recognition of the need to seek senior advice in the case of a serious incident. For more information on reporting concerns, refer back to Chapter 5.

B. *Filling in a CAE form* is the most appropriate response, because it will put in place a system that should prevent future thefts. Filling in the form needs to be done at the time of the incident and not retrospectively.

E. *Reporting the incident to the foundation director* is the next most appropriate option as this should help prevent future recurrence. Your foundation director will also be able to offer you advice on what you should do next. Remember, no matters which involve breaking confidentiality are ever urgent.

A. *Giving over the names of the patients so that you can make a claim* is the next most appropriate option. Although this does involve disclosing patient information, it would be justifiable, given the circumstances and having sought advice from a senior. You are not expected to put up with having your phone stolen

D. *Ignoring the situation and replacing your phone* is not appropriate. You are not expected to put up with theft and therefore this option – while in reality it may seem less complicated – is not what you **should** do.

C. *Accusing patients you suspect and questioning them about it* is the least appropriate response. This could produce potential distrust between you and your patients creating a potentially difficult situation for yourself.

---

7. A 16-year-old girl comes into A&E with diabetic ketoacidosis (DKA). She is admitted and treated. The following morning you are arranging her discharge. You discuss her diabetic control with her. She says that she can't be bothered with the insulin as it's too much hassle. What *should* you do?

ANSWER: BEACD

This question is asking you to consider your opportunities for learning. An FY1 should be willing to learn from others and from their experiences.

B. *Arranging for the diabetic specialist nurse to see her* is the most appropriate option, as they will have a wealth of experience with non-compliance and may have some tricks up their sleeve to deal with the situation. Ideally, you should utilise their skills and expertise by sitting in on their consultation so the nurse can educate you at the same time. This is the type of experience you may choose to reflect on in your eportfolio afterwards.

E. *Asking her why the insulin is such a problem* is the next most appropriate option. Is it because she can't do the same things as her friends? Or maybe she has a problem with her insulin regimen? Information means you can seek advice for a more suitable treatment plan.

A. *Educating her on the importance of compliance* is the next most appropriate, as it is your duty to inform patients of their responsibility for their own health. You should use every available opportunity you can for health promotion. The specialist diabetic nurse, of course, would do this for you as part of their consultation.

C. *Making a note of her non-compliance on the discharge summary to the GP* is the next most appropriate option. The GP should be made aware of the issue so that it can be followed up.

D. *Asking her parents to speak to her about compliance* is the least appropriate option as – given her age – you should try to engage with the patient first, rather than relying on her parents. You should still speak to her parents though, as they may also need educating about compliance. It would be best practice to let the girl know that you would like to speak to her parents about this. If there were circumstances in which she disagreed, you should seek senior advice from your consultant or registrar.

---

8. A 32-year-old woman presents to A&E for a head laceration. She claims that her boyfriend hit her, and she fell and hit her head. You smell alcohol on her breath. On questioning you find that she has left her two children at home under the supervision of her boyfriend who has also been drinking. You are worried about the children, what *should* you do?

ANSWER: BEDAC

This question incorporates social services protocol and expects you to demonstrate awareness of boundaries of your own competence. An FY1 should readily seek help when required. Refer back to Chapter 2 for specific information regarding social services.

B. *Calling your registrar to discuss the case* is the most appropriate option, as you will need senior consultation for advice regarding social services. They will also be able to guide you as to how to discuss the matter with the mother.

E. *Telling the mother you are concerned about the children, given her injuries* is the next most appropriate option as you first need to explain the reasoning behind your concerns

D. *Telling the mother that it is protocol that you put in a referral to social services* is the next most appropriate option as you need to explain what you are going to do about your concerns. You should always try to inform the parent that you are putting in a referral to social services, unless you feel that the child will be put at risk if you do so. In either case you would bring in a senior.

A. *Calling social services* is the next most appropriate option, as they will be able to advise on the phone whether an urgent response is necessary – i.e. to call the police to the house – or whether a referral through the usual mechanism is necessary. Social Services are the experts in this situation; hence, they should be the ones dictating the action plan.

C. *Filling in a referral form for social services* is the least appropriate option. Any form should be filled in at the time of concern when all the relevant information can be collected; but in this complex case it should be done by a senior. Moreover, as there is an immediate concern, the phone call should be made before the form is completed. However, if this was a more "routine" case, then the phone call would not be necessary and you would simply consult with a senior about completing the form.

---

9. Mrs Smith is 53-year-old woman who suffered with heart failure for many years. She has expressed a wish to receive no further treatment and go home to rest in peace. The nurse comes to see you the following day, saying that her husband has arrived and is angry that you are sending her home to die. He feels his wife is "out of her mind and not thinking straight". What *should* you do?

ANSWER: CAEBD

This question is about responding to a difficult situation between a patient and their relatives and respecting the wishes of both parties. An FY1 should understand both the relatives' and the patient's views for effective communication. See Chapter 4 for more advice on effective communication.

C. *Exploring the husband's concerns* is the most appropriate thing to do. This is because it is important as far as possible to respect the feelings of those close to the patient and meet their needs for support.

A. *Going to see Mrs Smith* is the next appropriate option, as you must find out whether her wish to refuse treatment is still the same. Moreover, you must gain consent to discuss Mrs Smith's wishes with her husband.

E. *Persuading Mrs Smith to go with you to speak to her husband about her wishes* follows on from A, as there is an opportunity for conflict resolution if both parties communicate their wishes to one another. This should be done once you have obtained consent.

B. *Asking the nurse to inform the husband it is Mrs Smith's decision* is not really appropriate. While it is possible for team members to resolve this issue, ideally it should be the person with the best rapport. Nurses have a great deal of communication with patients and their relatives and it is likely they've approached you because they feel out of their depth. You should appreciate the delicacy of this matter; simply directing the nurse without exploring the issue further is not appropriate.

D. *Referring Mrs Smith to psychiatry* is the least appropriate option as there is no indication that Mrs Smith needs psychiatric assessment, nor of it being any benefit to her.

---

10. Your FY1 colleague Mark has turned up late again for handover, and you smell alcohol on his breath. You know he has been having some family problems recently. You suspect the alcohol is from last night, but you cannot be sure. What *should* you do?

ANSWER: CDEBA

This question is about recognising and reporting dangerous practice. An FY1 should challenge unacceptable behaviour that threatens patient safety. Refer back to Chapter 5 for more information on reporting concerns.

C. *Suggesting to Mark that he explain the situation to the registrar* is the most appropriate option. This reduces the immediate risk to patient safety as the registrar can suggest the appropriate actions to take. This is an urgent situation as there is a potential compromise for patient care. However, you might not want to go straight to the consultant (D), as issues like this will affect your colleague's reputation. It is best if Mark can be persuaded to report his irresponsible behaviour.

D. *Reporting the situation immediately to your consultant* is the next most appropriate option. You have a responsibility to your patients, and your duty of care to them overrides your loyalty to your colleague. Serious incidents should immediately be raised, if they compromise patient safety. You are not in a position to deal with them yourself, so seniors must get involved.

E. *Having a quiet word with Mark after the handover* is the next most appropriate option, as you should offer your colleague the chance of an explanation and find out more about the situation. It is important that you support your colleagues, but having this conversation would not directly influence the outcome of the scenario as you should address the issue of patient safety first and foremost.

B. *Asking your education supervisor for advice* is the next most appropriate option. Getting confidential advice on clinical dilemmas should be considered, but this action will not address the immediate problem. You should consult those in your immediate team before more external clinicians. Although your educational supervisor will be at your hospital, it may take time to contact them.

A. *Reporting Mark immediately to the foundation programme director* is not appropriate. Reporting procedure is well outlined, and it is not your place to report this directly to the foundation programme director. They would expect you to go through the appropriate channels and try locally first. Moreover, the foundation director may not be on site and may take considerable time to respond which may result in a compromise in patient care. Your foundation programme director would eventually hear about it via the Doctors in Difficulty referral pathway.

---

11. An elderly woman is brought in by ambulance to A&E. She doesn't speak English. The paramedics say that she was found collapsed on the street and a passer-by called 999. She is stable, but you suspect she needs to be kept in overnight. You name some languages and she nods at "Urdu". It is 7.30 p.m., what *should* you do?

ANSWER: EDABC

This question includes a common problem with translation services and tests whether you can demonstrate initiative. Refer back to Chapter 4 for more information on working with interpreters.

E. *Finding a colleague on the ward to see if they can translate* is the most appropriate option. Whilst it is not an ideal solution, doctors and nurses remain impartial translators, and this means that you can get any urgent information from the patient while arranging for a more formal translator. Moreover, Urdu is a common language, and the likelihood of finding someone in the hospital who speaks it is high. Telephone services (e.g. language line) are expensive and should be considered as the next option if your colleagues cannot help.

D. *Arranging for a telephone interpretation* is the next appropriate option, as most A&E departments should have access to this service as arranged by the foundation trust. This service allows access to interpreters anytime, day or night and offers impartiality and confidentiality.

A. *Arranging for an interpreter to come to the hospital* is the next most appropriate option. No matter where you are working, the likelihood of getting an interpreter at 7.30 p.m. is slim. You could, however, leave a message and arrange this for the following morning. Typically, bilingual services are only available from 9 a.m.–5 p.m.

B. *Using an online translation service* would require a computer nearby that allows access to this service. It also requires that you type in the information, which is time-consuming. Moreover, there are limited languages available, and there is no guarantee that the translation is accurate. These services are generally inadequate for anything beyond the most basic of needs.

C. *Seeing if the patient can contact a friend or relative to interpret* is not appropriate. The use of an ad hoc interpreter is discouraged, and even more so if they have a close relationship with the patient. This option should be avoided where at all possible.

---

12. You are working on an oncology ward. It is a Saturday night, and a patient is asking you for the results of his myeloma screen. The nurse tells you that the patient is going to complain if they do not get the results soon. The patient is anxious and cannot understand why it is taking so long. You do not have their results yet. What *should* you do?

This question assesses your honesty and integrity with regard to the patient relationship and ensures that you make the patient your first concern.

E. *Apologising to the patient for the delay* is the most appropriate response – and also the most honest. By apologising you are showing empathy and acknowledging the patient's distress.

D. *Calling the registrar to speak to the patient* is the next most appropriate response, as this is a delicate issue that should be dealt with by a senior colleague.

A. *Explaining to the patient they are unlikely to get the results before Monday* is the next most appropriate response. This is an honest answer, but does not acknowledge the patient's concerns. It would be more appropriate to have a senior review the situation than to provide an inadequate explanation – especially when there has been the threat of a complaint.

C. *Calling the laboratory to put an urgent on the results* is the next most appropriate option, but this is unlikely to make any immediate difference to the situation as it is the weekend and other more urgent results will take priority.

B. *Telling the nurse to explain the delay to the patient* is not appropriate. It is important that you go and see the patient yourself and explain the situation. It is likely that the patient is threatening to make a complaint because they are worried. Hence, they will appreciate you taking the time to see them, helping to ease their anxiety.

---

13. You are working on a respiratory ward. A locum consultant prescribes antibiotics for Mr Jones for community-acquired pneumonia. You know these particular antibiotics are outside hospital guidelines. What *should* you do?

This question analyses your consideration for hospital policy and your ability to negotiate it with colleagues in an appropriate manner.

B. *Showing the guidelines to the consultant to ask whether they should be prescribed* is the most appropriate option as this addresses the issue and considers the options for prescribing.

C. *Asking the consultant the reasons for prescribing those antibiotics* is the next most appropriate option, because it may be that the consultant is aware of the guidelines but has prescribed them for a particular reason. Alternatively, these may be the ones that he typically uses, in which case you could enter into a discussion about local guidelines.

E. *Ringing pharmacy to find out their recommendations* is more appropriate than A or D. Pharmacy are an excellent source of guidance on the appropriate prescribing of medications. You should consult expert advice rather than either brush aside your concerns or undermine a colleague.

A. *Prescribing the treatment the consultant wishes outside guidelines* without good reason is not appropriate, as you should not ignore a situation where you think something is wrong. However, it is more appropriate to follow your consultant's wishes than to undermine their expertise and not carry out their management plan (D).

D. *Following the guidelines and ignoring the consultant's prescription* is the least appropriate option, as this means going against the advice of the consultant. If the patient were to deteriorate after you ignored their advice, you would be held soley responsible.

---

14. You are working a night shift on a surgical ward. A patient already on treatment for sepsis starts to rapidly deteriorate. It is nearly midnight. You complete your A to E primary survey and the patient is stable for the moment, but you feel you are out of your depth. You call the surgical registrar, but they tell you to call the medical team because they are busy in theatre. When you bleep the on-call medical

registrar, they tell you it is not their responsibility and to find someone else. What *should* you do?

Patient safety is always a first priority. It is important that you recognise your limitations and seek appropriate support when necessary. This should ideally be someone more experienced than yourself.

C. *Calling the surgical registrar again* is the most appropriate option, as they should give you the appropriate advice regarding immediate management steps that can be taken.

B. *Starting basic management for the patient* is the next most appropriate option, as you should take initial steps such as ordering investigations, taking bloods, prescribing fluids etc. as part of your secondary survey. These steps are within your remit, and you should optimise the care you can give in this situation.

D. *Asking a nurse to arrange for someone to help you* is the next most appropriate option as this involves sharing responsibility for the patient. The nurses are perfectly equipped to seek help for you while you attend to the patient. Moreover, they will have knowledge of who else could be contacted in this situation – for example, the hospital may have a critical care outreach team. However, this is less appropriate than informing seniors, as it does not directly address patient care. Moreover, you have more knowledge of the patient's clinical condition and it is better to relay this information yourself.

A. Although *calling the consultant at home is not a nice thing to have to do*, it is perfectly acceptable and would be the next appropriate action if no seniors were available on site. They will, however, be 20, 30 minutes away from the hospital . . . maybe more. The patient, at the end of the day, comes first and as the consultant's responsibility overall, he/she would rather be contacted regarding problems with patient care.

E. *Putting out a periarrest call on 2222* is not appropriate, as the question clearly says that the patient is stable. This should only be used if you feel the patient is going to arrest. Think of calling 2222 like dialling 999: for instance you would think twice about calling if someone in a restaurant looked very well and was simply having heartburn rather than having a heart attack.

---

15. A patient with end-stage motor neurone disease asks you to give them the lethal injection. You explain to them that this is not legal in this country. What *should* you do?

This question explores patient focus. An FY1 is expected to appreciate needs, build relationships with patients, be respectful of patients' wishes and work in partnership about their care. However, FY1s are not expected to follow patient's wishes when it involves euthanasia!

A. *Exploring the patient's reasons for wanting the lethal injection* is the most appropriate option, because it is important that you find out from the patient whether it is due to depression or whether they are trying to convey specific preferences about their treatment.

E. *Explaining to the patient about an advance directive* is the next most appropriate option, as you would highlight the choices available to them concerning their treatment.

C. *Asking the patient to talk to their partner about their feelings* may result in them getting additional advice and support if they so wish. This response, however, would not address the immediate issue.

D. *Referring the patient to psychiatry* is not appropriate, as it is not clear that the patient has a mental health issue. You would also need senior input before making this decision.

B. *Telling the patient's partner how they feel* is the least appropriate option as you would be breaking patient confidentiality.

---

16. An 83-year-old man is brought in to A&E after a fall. He has severe dementia and is obviously in pain, but is unable to tell you where the pain is coming from. After examination you suspect he has a broken hip. This is confirmed by X-ray. A decision needs to be made about treatment. However, he lacks capacity. His wife is deceased and his daughter, detailed as his next of kin, lives in Australia. What *should* you do?

This question tests your knowledge of consent where a patient does not have capacity in an emergency situation. Refer to Chapter 5 for more information.

E. *Starting treatment* is the most appropriate option, as the patient comes first, and you do not need consent to give analgesia – this is a basic treatment option that provides overall benefit for a patient in pain.

C. *Speaking to the registrar about scheduling him onto the surgical list* is the next most appropriate option. The responsibility for decisions about treatment in an emergency situation lies with the treating doctors. Emergency treatment must be provided straight away. A senior needs to be made aware of the situation ASAP as a broken hip can be potentially life-threatening. Although it would not be your responsibility to schedule a patient onto the surgical list, this option directly advocates for treatment of the patient by directly involving their care.

A. *Contacting your local IMCA* is the next most appropriate option. Typically, an IMCA is appointed in non-emergency situations where a family member or friend cannot be contacted. This service advocates for patients who lack capacity to ensure that their feelings and wishes are considered. As broken hips are scheduled onto the trauma list, this is an emergency situation; however, as the patient has severe dementia, they will be useful for assistance in less pressing matters. It is, therefore, appropriate to contact them early in case a difficult decision has to be made post-surgery.

D. *Checking through the notes for any legal documentation* is the next most appropriate thing to do, as this will give you an idea of the patient's wishes as well as any documents detailing a legal proxy whom you could contact to make his decisions for him. Although this will be useful in informing decisions, a thorough search should not prevent emergency treatment and this could take some time given his age and co-morbidities.

B. *Trying to contact his daughter in Australia* is the least appropriate option. Whilst you should contact a patient's relatives and close friends when trying to make a decision about "overall benefit", they do not have the final say in treatment. You can assume that the patient would want them involved if they lack capacity, but again this is different when the situation is an emergency. This would not change your management of the patient and is therefore the last action you would take in this situation.

---

17. It is a quiet afternoon on your surgical ward. The consultant asks you to come and assist with a private list in the afternoon at a different hospital. What *should* you do?

ANSWER: CDAEB

This question is about juggling your work commitments with opportunities for career progression.

C. *Declining and going to assist in theatres* is the most appropriate option, as you should utilise quiet times on the ward to seek out additional learning opportunities. This option is appropriate and enhances your educational development. Whilst it is not appropriate to leave the hospital, it is perfectly acceptable to seek experiences on site and, as a trainee, you should be taking advantage of such situations.

D. *Declining because you have responsibilities on the ward* is the next most appropriate option, as this immediately addresses the issue. Whilst this would be a good opportunity, you should not leave the hospital during paid working time. It would not be fair to your colleagues to increase their workload. Nor would it be fair to your patients whose care may suffer as a result. If you explained this to the consultant, they should understand this.

A. *Asking your education supervisor* is the next most appropriate option as you should ask for senior advice when faced with a dilemma. Moreover, educational supervisors should be in your hospital; therefore, you should receive a timely response from them.

E. Should you not be able to contact your educational supervisor, *seeking advice from a fellow FY1* is the next most appropriate response. Although they won't have the same level of expertise, they may have faced a similar situation, or know someone else who has.

B. *Agreeing to help your consultant with the private list* is the least appropriate option as it is unacceptable to leave without formally handing over patients. Moreover, it is not appropriate to leave your patients while you are being paid by the NHS to care for them – no matter how quiet the ward is!

---

18. You are seeing a patient in minors in A&E on a Friday night. A nurse comes in to tell you that a patient is being verbally aggressive and threatening because they haven't been seen yet and thinks people are "jumping the queue". The nurse suspects the patient has been drinking alcohol. What *should* you do?

ANSWER: BDACE

Nurses handle a great deal on the wards. If they come to see you about an aggressive patient, they will likely have tried everything to calm them down, so be sympathetic.

B. *Asking the nurse to call security* is the most appropriate option. Staff are not expected to tolerate abuse and calling security is a necessary precaution as there is a potential for this situation to get worse. Security can act quickly if it does escalate.

D. *Explaining to the patient you are busy but will see them as soon as possible* is the next most appropriate option, as patients will often calm down if given a rational explanation.

A. *Going to see the patient and telling them they will not be treated unless they calm down* is more appropriate than C and E. However, a patient's right to treatment should never be influenced by their behaviour, and the GMC recommends that you do not use treatment as a bargaining power.

C. *Telling the nurse to get someone else to see the patient* is not appropriate. You might be the only person that the nurse could find to help. If you did nothing and something were to happen to the nurse because there was no one else around, then you would be held accountable. This would be an error in judgement. You should prioritise this situation as more urgent than the patient you are seeing to in minors, as there is a potential for harm.

E. *Physically restraining the patient* is the least appropriate option. You cannot physically restrain a patient without just cause, as restraint may be considered physical assault. This would be the role of security.

---

19. A 60-year-old Indian man comes into A&E with a history of fits. He was discharged 2 days ago from ITU. His wife is with him, but she does not speak English. He is very confused, disorientated and, from your A to E assessment, clearly unwell. You cannot get a history. It is 4 p.m. on a Monday afternoon. What *should* you do?

ANSWER: ADBEC

This question is about prioritisation and problem-solving. An FY1 should demonstrate initiative when it comes to information gathering and think creatively to solve problems.

A. *Proceeding anyway with routine examination and investigations* is the most appropriate option as you must rule out anything potentially life-threatening before you get more information on this patient's history. You can obtain a lot of information from examination alone. It is not acceptable to neglect examining a patient just because you can't get a good history. Patient care is your clinical priority and should always be done first. If needs be, he can be treated as a new patient rather than as a failed discharge.

D. *Asking ITU to fax over the notes from the previous admission* is the next most appropriate option, as this will give you access to the notes quickly – if they have them. They also might have information on the patient's family, translators, etc.

B. *Ringing the GP to get background information* is the next most appropriate option. The GP should be the first port of call for patient information. In this case, however, the GP may not have the most recent information on the patient, given that it is only two days since discharge and it typically takes longer for discharge information to be received. Don't be alarmed if the GP asks to call you back on your bleep, or to fax the notes over – this should be standard protocol to protect patient confidentiality.

E. *Arranging for an interpreter* is the next most appropriate option. However, interpreters take time to arrange and it is unlikely that you will get one within an hour. This situation is potentially urgent and therefore other options should be explored in preference to this.

C. *Ringing the patient's family* is the least appropriate option. This would break confidentiality and there is no guarantee that they speak English either. His wife is already present with whom the interpreter could consult.

---

20. You are working as an FY1 on an obstetrics and gynaecology ward. A 29-year-old woman is admitted 4 hours into labour. This is her first pregnancy. She is requesting a Caesarean section (CS), but there is no medical indication for it at this stage. This is different from her birth plan, but the patient is demanding that she be given the care that she wants. What *should* you do?

This question is about working in partnership with patients about their care whilst bearing in mind their best interests. In terms of a patient's best interests concerning a CS, indications for a CS include (NICE 2011):
- Presumed foetal compromise
- 'Failure to progress' in labour
- Breech presentation (~10% of all CS)
- Placenta praevia
- Multiple pregnancy

When a woman requests a CS NICE (2011) recommends:
- Discussing the overall risks and benefits of a CS and vaginal birth, taking into account circumstances, concerns and priorities
- Including a discussion with other members of the obstetric team (obstetrician, midwife and anaesthetist) to explore reasons for a request and to ensure the woman has the accurate information
- Offering perinatal mental health support for women with anxiety about childbirth
- If this is unsuccessful, offering a planned CS with a willing obstetrician. If the consultant obstetrician is not willing, the team should refer to one who is.

C. *Exploring the patient's reasons for wanting a CS* is the most appropriate option. This demonstrates consideration for their needs and is the first step towards reaching a solution.

B. *Ringing the consultant obstetrician* is the next most appropriate option as they will be making the final decision and need to be made aware of the situation as soon as it arises. You will also be able to discuss with them over the phone the risks and benefits of both a CS and vaginal birth (D), which you could relay to the patient before the consultant arrives.

D. *Explaining the overall risks and benefits of a CS and vaginal birth* is the next most appropriate option. NICE (2011) recommends this is carried out before any decision is made regarding a CS. If the patient still wants to change her birth plan at this point, then you have already appropriately informed your seniors.

A. *Asking the midwife on the ward for advice* is the next most appropriate option. The midwife is part of the obstetric team and will undoubtedly have dealt with this situation before. However, they would not make a final decision for this patient, and therefore you should approach an obstetrician in preference in this case.

E. *Refusing the CS* is the least appropriate option. This patient has a right to a CS regardless of whether it is medically indicated, and you are not in a position to refuse such treatment to this patient.

---

21. A 27-year old woman comes into A&E with vomiting and mild abdominal pain. You have sent off bloods, but in the meantime the routine pregnancy test comes back positive. Her fiancé rings casualty to ask how she is doing. What *should* you do?

This question is about patient confidentiality. Refer to Chapter 2 for more information on confidentiality breaches.

D. *Telling her partner that you will need to get her consent before you tell him anything* is the most appropriate option, as you must respect patient confidentiality. Generally, members of the public understand this and will appreciate your honesty. This option immediately resolves the issue.

C. *Telling her partner that he will have to speak to his fiancée directly* is the next most appropriate response, as you are respecting confidentiality whilst being honest with her fiancée.

E. *Telling her partner that you are still waiting for the results of all the investigations* is the next most appropriate option, as this does not involve giving the fiancé false reassurance (*see* B). Although this woman is pregnant, there could also be other explanations for her symptoms which you would want to exclude before she was discharged. You are not being dishonest with this explanation, as there are bloods pending.

B. *Telling her partner that it is nothing serious and that she will be fine* is less appropriate, given that you cannot confidently make this claim. This however is more appropriate than A – actually breaking confidentiality.

A. *Telling her partner that she is pregnant* is not appropriate. You do not have the patient's consent to reveal this information, and this would break patient confidentiality.

22. You are an FY1 working on a gastroenterology ward. A nurse comes to tell you that one of the patients with chronic alcoholism has been very rude. This is not the first time it has happened. The nurse is clearly quite upset, what *should* you do?

ANSWER: ABEDC

This scenario involves prioritising your colleague's needs over the patients by offering them your support.

A. *Telling the nurse you will speak to the patient* is the most appropriate option, as this shows your colleague that you take their complaint seriously whilst giving the patient the opportunity to express their own opinion on the situation. There are two sides to every story and it is best to elicit them before intervening.

B. *Going to speak to the patient* is the next most appropriate option, as abuse towards the staff should not to be tolerated and the patient should be made aware of this. This option also allows you to find out the patient's reasons for acting in the manner the nurse described.

E. *Asking the patient to apologise to the nurse* is the next most appropriate option. Out of respect to the nurse, it would be polite to request that the patient apologise.

D. *Advising the nurse to work in a different section* is not appropriate, as it does not directly address the problem. It will be difficult for the nurse just to ignore part of the ward when resources are already stretched. Moreover, this patient's behaviour may extend to abusing other members of the team, which is unacceptable.

C. *Advising the nurse to ignore it* is the least appropriate option as the question clearly states that this isn't the first time it has happened. Moreover, your colleague is upset; staff are not expected to tolerate abuse in any form.

23. A patient – well known to psychiatry – is admitted onto the gastro ward with a history of somatisation disorder (multiple physical complaints with a psychological cause). She is demanding a bowel resection following a colonoscopy. The results of the colonoscopy are completely normal and surgery is not clinically indicated. She is angry that you will not treat her and threatens to "cut it out herself if you don't". What *should* you do?

ANSWER: DCEBA

This question is about responding appropriately to a difficult patient with a mental health issue.

D. *Explaining to the patient you think this is part of their mental health problem* is the most appropriate option. You are explaining honestly the reasons for not operating. Moreover, it may help calm the patient if you show that you have taken them seriously, but that you are aware of their condition. You can also assess the patient at this point to see how unwell they are.

C. *Reiterating to the patient that you cannot operate because the colonoscopy was normal* is the next most appropriate option. Repeating honestly why you cannot operate makes sure you are consistent in your explanation.

E. *Calling the senior registrar for advice* is the next most appropriate option. This is a difficult patient, and there is a potential for serious harm should she act on her threats. You should recognise that this is beyond your remit and seek help accordingly. The registrar will also be able to advise you on how to manage this patient further and on any other explanations you can give to try and calm the patient down.

B. *Bleeping the on-call psychiatrist* is the next most appropriate option. As the patient is already known to psychiatry, you should seek their opinion, particularly given the serious threat of self-harm. Following psychiatric assessment she may need admitting to a psychiatric unit where she can receive alternative care.

A. *Agreeing with the patient she can have surgery if she calms down* is the least appropriate option as under no circumstances should you lie to a patient. This would have disastrous consequences for the patient's mental health: never bargain treatments with patients.

24. You are working as an FY1 in a GUM clinic. You are seeing a young man with newly diagnosed Hepatitis B. He is an ex-intravenous drug user who works in a bar. You question him about his partner and discover that he has not disclosed his Hepatitis B status as he is afraid this will mean his partner will leave him. He says they are having protected sexual intercourse. What *should* you do?

ANSWER: CADEB

This question requires you respect patient confidentiality. In the case of communicable diseases the GMC recommends (GMC 2009f):

• You should tell the patient that you will share their information with those in the immediate healthcare team involved in their care – unless they object.

• You cannot force a patient to reveal their infection status unless someone is at risk of infection.

• You should explain to the patient how to minimise infection risk to others.

• As with any issue, you can disclose information without consent if justifiable e.g. serious harm.

• When tracing contacts, identity should not be revealed.

For more information on confidentiality see Chapter 2.

C. *Explaining you have to duty to tell his partner about their risk of infection* is the most appropriate option, as this response most directly considers the safety of his partner without putting the patient in a more difficult situation. You have a legal requirement to disclose the information to the person at risk (GMC 2009f). It is also recommended that you tell the patient before you make any disclosures and reiterate that they will **not** be identified in the process.

A. *Trying to persuade him to tell his partner* is the next most appropriate response, as the GMC (2009f) recommends that you make every effort to persuade infectious patients to inform those at risk. Given the hesitancy in this scenario, however, it is unlikely that you will change his mind, and patients cannot be forced into disclosing their diagnosis. It is therefore your responsibility rather than the patient's to ensure that information is shared.

D. *Offering to talk to the patient and his partner together* is the next most appropriate option, as offering your support may be all that is necessary for the patient to agree to disclosure. This will relieve some of his pressure, as many patients find breaking bad news extremely challenging. Lending an expert opinion could make all the difference.

E. *Recommending counselling* is the next most appropriate option. This should have been offered at time of diagnosis but the scenario suggests they may be having difficulties coping with the issue.

B. *Not disclosing information because there is "no risk"* is the least appropriate option. As mentioned above, there is a potential risk to the partner, and you have a duty to protect them, as well as a duty to the patient.

---

25. You are an FY1 working on a labour ward. One of your patients has a breech presentation. She has a birth plan which specifies that every appropriate method should be attempted before opting for a Caesarean section. She has now changed her mind and decided to have a CS. Her husband disagrees; taking you to one side and saying "she's in pain, she doesn't know what she wants, she'll regret it if you operate". What *should* you do?

This question is about managing contrasting views of patients and their relatives, necessitating good communication skills. An FY1 is expected to adapt their style of communication according to the context.

D. *Reminding him that this is his wife's choice* is the most appropriate option. You should respect the opinions of relatives, but, at the end of the day, decisions about treatment should always be made by the patient (provided they have capacity).

C. *Enquiring into her reasons for the change in birth plan* is the next most appropriate option. You can then communicate this to your consultant. It is best practice to get as much information on the case before seeking senior advice.

B. *Calling the consultant obstetrician to review the patient* is the next most appropriate option, as this is a decision above your level; hence you need help. The situation is relatively

urgent given the potential risk to the mother and the unborn child. The consultant will also be able to advise you on how to best proceed with management in the interim.

A. *Informing the patient about a CS and vaginal birth* is the next most appropriate option, as the patient needs to be aware of the risks and benefits for both procedures. It is likely that she will have been over this in her birth plan. However, it is important to cover this again before any decisions are made.

E. *Asking the husband to leave so you can speak to the patient in private* is the least appropriate option. This removes the support of her husband and could potentially cause more distress to the patient. Also, the consultant would make a decision whether the patient was being coerced by her husband or not. You should try to maintain harmony in this scenario and removing the husband is not the way forward.

---

26. You are working on a gastroenterology ward and a nurse approaches you and says Mr Brown needs to be prescribed his usual fluids. You are finishing up a discharge summary and take home drugs for another patient. What *should* you do?

This question requires you to consider prescribing errors and patient safety in a pressured environment. An FY1 is expected to remain calm when under pressure, demonstrate good judgement and manage uncertainty. Refer to Chapter 3 for more information on safe prescribing and prioritisation.

E. *Asking about Mr Brown's fluid status* is the most appropriate option. You need to find out more information from the nurse about Mr Brown before you can make an educated decision about the urgency of this task. For example, if the nurse was concerned about a low urine output, you might go and see him straight away. If there was no concern, then you would finish the prescription and see him afterwards. You should always prioritise tasks according to clinical need.

D. *To say you will put it on your jobs list and get to it as soon as you can* is the next most appropriate option as this means you can prioritise it accordingly. Discharge summaries are important and involve prescribing and dosages. You should not be distracted from this task if possible as it may mean that the patient is discharged without the appropriate medications, or on the wrong medication etc.

C. *Explaining that to enable you to get the discharges done they should ask another FY1* is an abrupt response, but prioritising the discharge summaries over this routine prescription is more appropriate than (B) or (A). You should be supportive towards colleagues, but recognise when to say no. Moreover, the nurses and ward clerks are under pressure to discharge patients and they should understand your reasons.

B. *Going to see Mr Brown straight away* is a less appropriate option. In this case, the priority of care is ensuring that the patient you are discharging gets the right medication and has the relevant information communicated to their GP. There is no indication in this scenario that Mr Brown is unwell and therefore his "usual" fluids can wait.

A. *Prescribing Mr Brown his normal saline* is the least appropriate option, as this is potentially dangerous. If you overload Mr Brown with fluid you could cause pulmonary oedema. Always remember to see the patient before you prescribe in order to minimise error.

---

27. A colleague has left 30 minutes early to attend a dental appointment. They have asked you to prescribe Warfarin for their patient. Your shift has already ended, and you were about to go home. The INR result from the morning's blood tests is not back yet. What *should* you do?

This question is about safe prescribing and prioritising patient care. Refer to Chapter 3 for information on pressures, prescribing and prioritisation.

E. *Ringing the lab to see if the INR results are available* is the most appropriate option, as you should find out why the results have taken so long. It may be that the sample has been missed off, in which case you would need to rebleed the patient – or ask them if they can do a repeat. Usually the lab will save part of the sample for such cases. Whilst you are not expected to stay long after your shift has ended, you have accepted responsibility for this patient and therefore you should make their care a priority before you leave.

B. *Handing over the request to the ward cover* is the next most appropriate option, as you should make sure that the patient has a continuation of care and receives their Warfarin in a safe manner.

D. *Recording that the patient needs their Warfarin dosing in the notes* is the next most appropriate option. Although writing in the notes does not ensure that it will get done, having a record means you can check it in the morning. Not having the patient's Warfarin dosed could be equally as detrimental as overprescribing it. It is always good practice to write in the notes as well as make a personal list.

C. *Writing it onto your job list for the morning* is the next most appropriate option, as you should make a note to yourself to check that this has been done. After all, this patient is now your responsibility.

A. *Prescribing the Warfarin anyway* is not appropriate, as prescribing this without the INR result potentially puts the patient at risk of bleeding.

---

28. You are working as an FY1 on a surgical ward. On your way to ordering a CT scan from radiology you are bleeped. You find the nearest phone to ring through. A nurse is concerned about Mrs Fazi's urine output (UO). You remember it was fine for her small frame when you checked two hours ago. What *should* you do?

This question is about coping with pressure. An FY1 is expected to adapt to changing circumstances and manage uncertainty. They should also be able to re-prioritise tasks as necessary.

D. *Asking the nurse whether Mrs Fazi's UO has changed since this morning* is the most appropriate option as you need to find out more about Mrs Fazi before you can make a decision.

A. *Asking the nurse to do some basic observations whilst you order the CT* is the next most appropriate option as you need to get scans approved early in the day for them to get done. The scan is, therefore, prioritised as urgent. Not completing this task may cause that patient to suffer. Your consultant will not be impressed if you don't get the scan, as it will mess up the patient's management plan.

C. *Reassuring the nurse that Mrs Fazi's UO was fine for her size* is the next most appropriate option, as it may be that the nurse hasn't accounted for her small frame. If it was fine two hours ago, you can reassure the nurse that it is sensible to order the CT scan first before going to check on Mrs Fazi.

B. *Going to see Mrs Fazi immediately* is not appropriate. You should not drop everything when there is no indication that there is an emergency. You should address the nurse's concerns in a timely manner, whilst making sure that you prioritise effectively. It is better to spend 15 minutes ordering a CT scan and attend to Mrs Fazi after.

E. *Telling the nurse to start fluids* is not appropriate, as you should not prescribe over the phone, nor should you prescribe for a patient that you haven't been to see yourself.

---

29. You go to see a patient with whom you previously had trouble putting in a cannula. You ask them whether you can take some blood. They recognise you and say "don't come anywhere near me with that thing, you don't know what you're doing". What *should* you do?

This question is about taking responsibility for your own actions and owning up to mistakes.

A. *Reassuring the patient that you are competent at taking blood* is the most appropriate option as you should reassure the patient of your clinical skills. This response directly addresses the situation.

C. *Apologising to the patient for yesterday* is the next most appropriate option, as you need to show the patient that you accept responsibility for causing them distress. The patient may also be more likely to consent to venepuncture on acceptance of your apology. This, however, would be best after some reassurance of your ability.

B. *Asking a nurse to take their blood* is the next most appropriate option, as you should not lie to force the patient to consent (D) and you cannot take blood from the cannula (E) as it will

be contaminated. Although nurses are busy, they can always help you out and some will be trained in taking blood.

D. *Telling the patient that you have to take their blood because there is no-one else* is not appropriate. This is coercing the patient to consent. You should attempt to find someone else to take it before you tell them that they have no other options.

E. *Taking blood from their cannula* is not appropriate. There are few occasions when you can take blood from a cannula as fluids and drugs will have passed through it. The sample would be contaminated, which means the lab would process the bloods erroneously.

---

30. A patient you recently discharged from the ward requests your friendship on a social networking site. They are a similar age to you. What *should* you do?

This question is about professionalism. For advice on social networking refer to Chapter 2.

B. *Declining the friend request and explaining your reasons* is the most appropriate option. The BMA (2011) recommends that you decline any offers of friendship and explain why to the patient. This most effectively addresses the problem.

E. *Asking your educational supervisor for advice* is the next most appropriate option, as they will be able to explain what to do in this situation and turn it into a learning experience. You gain more from this than you would from ignoring the situation and not seeking advice.

C. *Ignoring the request* is the next most appropriate option, as it is better to ignore a friend request than accept it. This would address the problem but not necessarily solve it. It would be more appropriate to learn from the experience by seeking advice.

D. *Asking your FY1 colleague for advice* is the next most appropriate option. Although this will not directly solve the issue, your colleagues should have an understanding of professionalism and best practice and may be able to give advice.

A. *Accepting the request* is not appropriate. It is not advisable to accept online friendships with patients or former patients. Irrespective of their discharge, they could at any point come under your care again, and it is unprofessional to enter into this kind of relationship.

---

31. You are working on ITU, completing the morning's jobs list. When taking bloods from a patient – admitted following a road traffic accident – you accidently stick yourself with the needle. You had followed infection control guidelines and were wearing gloves but you see your finger bleeding underneath. You quickly squeeze it, clean it and put a dressing on it. You go to look on the system for anything on the patient's HIV/Hepatitis status but there is nothing. The patient is unconscious. What *should* you do?

This question is asking whether you understand best practice following a stick injury.

B. *Ringing occupational health* is appropriate, as they will be able to tell you immediately the protocol for stick injuries.

D. *Filling in a CAE form* is appropriate, as when you go to occupational health, they will ask whether you have filled this in.

G. *Bleeping your registrar to explain the situation* is appropriate, as you will have to go to occupational health, thereby leaving ITU. You should always notify a senior of a serious incident – as in this case – so they can make the appropriate arrangements such that neither your own nor the patient's safety is compromised.

A. *Requesting viral serology* is not appropriate, as the patient has not consented to having these investigations and it would not be in their best interests to have them done. If they were in ITU for an illness in which HIV status could benefit their treatment, then this could be considered. You, however, would not request this; it would have to be done by a senior.

C. *Going to A&E for anti-retrovirals* is not appropriate during working hours. Occupational health will be able to give you the appropriate advice and treatment. If occupational health cannot be contacted, you should go to A&E where an appropriate risk assessment and management can be carried out.

E. *Asking if you can go home* is not appropriate, as this would be a way of avoiding, rather than helping, this situation.

F. *Waiting to see if the patient wakes up to ask for their permission for serology* is not appropriate. The patient is unconscious and therefore you have no idea when they will wake up. You should act quickly and promptly after a stick injury to reduce the risk to yourself as far as possible.

H. *Explaining to one of the nurses what has happened* is not a preferred option as you should inform your senior before the nurses. The nurse's priority is largely patient safety, whereas a senior colleague will be able to analyse the situation and manage the team to best support your needs and ensure the patient's best interests are considered.

---

32. Your FY1 colleague turns up late again for their shift. The ward you are working on is quiet. Your colleague arrives in tears; she is feeling exhausted, stressed and says that she is not coping with anything at the minute. This is the third time in the past two weeks. What *should* you do?

This is about supporting a doctor in difficulty and prioritising your colleagues.

B. *Sitting your colleague down to talk about her problems* is the most appropriate option. Your colleague is clearly distressed and therefore you should deal with this issue in a timely manner.

F. *Advising your colleague to talk to her educational supervisor* is also appropriate, as their supervisor should be the "go-to" person for support. They have access to the "doctors in difficulty" programme, if needed. It is always better that you flag up issues with your supervisor rather than ignoring them and letting them be referred in via a different avenue.

C. *Suggesting she book an appointment to see her GP* is an appropriate option. Although you don't yet know what is causing her stress, it might be good for her to talk to someone external without the added pressure of feeling judged by her seniors. GPs are also used to seeing patients with health problems caused by stress on a daily basis and will be able to recommend a sensible way forward – including recommending sick leave.

G. *Seeking advice from your educational supervisor* is not a preferred option. Although your educational supervisor is a good point of contact when you are unsure how to handle a situation, your supervisor can't do much to help your colleague if she has a different educational supervisor. Your educational supervisor could be helpful if you needed to debrief on how you handled the situation.

E. *Suggesting she take sick leave* will not address the issue and is therefore not appropriate. If it involves stress at work, taking leave will only prolong it until they return. Also her GP would be the most appropriate person to make this decision.

A. *Apologising and saying that you are busy* is not appropriate, given how upset your colleague is, and the question clearly states that you are on a quiet ward. Moreover, this isn't the first time she has displayed a significant amount of distress.

D. *Suggesting your colleague speak to her registrar* is not a preferred option. While she could speak to her registrar, it is sensible to seek advice from those in the best position to help.

H. *Mentioning that you have to inform your consultant of her difficulties* is not appropriate, as this may alienate your colleague further. As there is no indication of compromise to patient safety, you should be supportive rather than accusatory and recommend she seek help through the appropriate channels.

---

33. You are working in Children's A&E on a Saturday night. A 13-year-old boy comes in drunk. He admits he has been drinking alcohol and says he fell over. The X-ray confirms he has broken his index and middle fingers. The boy is adamant he is fine and doesn't want any treatment because he is scared that his parents will find out he has been drinking. He wants you to just give him some painkillers and then he'll leave. What *should* you do?

This question is asking you about acting in the patient's best interests for someone who does not have the capacity to refuse treatment. See Chapter 2 for more information on patient advocacy for the under eighteens.

H. *Discussing the situation with the nurse in charge* is appropriate, as the nurses on this unit will have experience in dealing with teenagers refusing treatment. They will be able to give you advice. They also might be able to talk to the boy and get him to stay.

E. *Trying to persuade him to have his fingers splinted* is appropriate, as you should make every effort to help this boy understand that he should have treatment. This is easier than having to force him to stay.

C. *Explaining that you really need to let his parents know what has happened and it would be best if he rang them* is appropriate, as this boy is a minor and has been drinking alcohol, and therefore is unlikely to be Gillick competent. He is also at risk of harm from further alcohol abuse and injury. If he self-discharged and his parents knew nothing about it, your professionalism could be questioned.

A. *Prescribing the painkillers and letting him self-discharge* is not appropriate. You should not prescribe pain relief if he has been drinking alcohol; moreover, it is in his best interests that he does not self-discharge.

B. *Ringing the boy's parents without telling him* is not appropriate, as this is breaking confidentiality. You should always inform the patient if you are going to do this.

D. *Telling him to go and see his GP if he has any problems over the weekend* is not appropriate, as he has not self-discharged yet.

F. *Putting in a referral for social services* is not appropriate at this stage as there is no need for intervention by social services on this evidence alone.

G. *Refusing to let him self-discharge without getting the proper treatment* is not a preferred option. A teenager can only consent to treatment; they cannot refuse treatment even if they are Gillick competent, as this must be overridden if you consider treatment to be in their best interests. It is, therefore, more appropriate to get senior support. Remember to select the options that are the most appropriate to your role as an FY1.

---

34. You are on a ward round with your consultant on the coronary care unit. The patient's relatives are sitting in the waiting room at the end of the corridor. Your consultant says that the patient is going to die soon and checks the Do Not Attempt Resuscitation (DNAR) form. The family approach you politely after the ward round whilst you are ordering bloods and say "so you think Mum is going to die, do you?" It is clear they have overheard your consultant's comments. What *should* you do?

This question considers how you deal with a difficult situation involving relatives. Remember that good communication is TPP: at the right Time, with the appropriate People in the appropriate Place.

H. *Calling your consultant to explain what has happened* is appropriate. This is a complex situation and your consultant really is the most appropriate person to deal with this matter. You can discuss with the consultant over the phone how you should proceed.

A. *Asking a nurse to take the family to a side room* is appropriate, as this is a sensitive issue that would best be approached in a neutral space. Moreover, as it is a potentially volatile situation, having a colleague for support is a good idea.

D. *Apologising to the family* is appropriate, as you will clearly have caused the relatives some distress in hearing about their mother in such frank terms. An apology demonstrates your sensitivity towards their needs.

F. *Asking the family if they would like to sit with their mother* is not a preferred option, given the nature of the situation. They should be directed to an appropriate room to await the consultant to have a detailed conversation. They may wish to sit with their relative after this time, but it would be best to have a discussion on neutral ground rather than at the bedside.

B. *Asking where they heard that information* is not appropriate, as it is obvious there has been error, irrespective of where they heard this information.

C. *Telling them you are busy* and **G.** *Finishing ordering the bloods* are not appropriate, as both actions are rude and do not appropriately deal with this situation. Bloods can wait for 20 minutes whilst this issue is addressed.

E. *Filling in a CAE form* is not a preferred option. This could be considered at a later stage after the incident has been managed appropriately. Also, the consultant may wish to complete the form in this case.

---

35. A nine-year-old boy was admitted following an exacerbation of asthma. You speak with the parents about using his steroid inhaler. The boy's mother is happy to make sure he has the inhaler; however, his father is clearly not. The father says that he has heard that they will stunt his boy's growth and he doesn't want that. What *should* you do?

This question is about acknowledging a parent's concerns and managing them appropriately to ensure compliance with medication which is in the best interests of your patient.

G. *Educating the father about the advantages of using an inhaler* is appropriate, as the father may have some misconceptions – in which case you can iron them out through education and help change his mind about the inhaler.

F. *Planning to monitor the boy's growth on a growth chart* is also appropriate, as this is addresses the concerns of the father by diligently monitoring for any side effects. By recording the boy's growth on the chart, you are showing that you take his misgivings seriously, which will hopefully improve compliance in the long term.

C. *Asking the asthma specialist nurse for advice* is another appropriate option, as it is likely the specialist nurse will have

dealt with a similar scenario before and may have some tricks to help handle the situation.

H. *Asking the boy what he would like to do* is not a preferred choice as although you should try to involve any child as much as possible in their care, acknowledging the parent's disagreement should be the priority. Moreover, this boy is only nine years old and too young to consent to treatment himself.

E. *Getting the mother to persuade the father* is not a preferred option as you must try to educate the father first, and get some more advice, before using the other parent as the mediator. The evidence of healthcare professionals should be much more effective than the mother's opinion alone. Moreover, this would not adequately address the father's concerns.

B. *Contacting social services about the disagreement* is not appropriate, as there is nothing to indicate that this child is at risk of harm.

D. *Agreeing with the father not to use the steroid inhaler* is not appropriate, as it would not be in the best interests of the child to stop his asthma medication.

A. *Ignoring the father's wishes* is not appropriate, as you should make every effort to resolve the dispute so that the child receives the same message from both parents. If they conflict, mixed messages can lead to increased non-compliance. Be careful not confuse the issue of consent with the issue of compliance. Although only one parent is needed to consent to treatment, in this case you want both parents on the same page so that the boy receives his medication in the appropriate manner.

---

36. A 43-year-old man is brought in by ambulance to A&E after collapsing in a bar on a Friday night. You have no details other than his name and date of birth, which the paramedics got from his wallet. The man is incapable of giving a history due to his level of intoxication. He is stable in the resuscitation area. What *should* you do?

This is about patient prioritisation in an emergency situation and recognising your job role and limitations. An FY1 should be proactive and able to initiate assessment and investigations but know when to seek help: in this case for starting treatment.

A. *Continuing with your A to E assessment* is appropriate, as you should always go back to basics for every patient.

G. *Starting the appropriate investigations but no new medications* is appropriate, as you must treat the patient as new if you don't know anything. You can hold off starting any medications until you have tried to find out whether he has any allergies or is on any medications that may interact.

C. *Asking a clerk to search the hospital database for any records* is appropriate. Patient care should be your priority, and finding more about his medications and past medical history is essential. A clerk should have time to look through the database and print off any old clinical letters to find out more about him.

B. *Ringing your registrar* is not a preferred option. You should complete your A to E assessment and then see what you can find out about his history. It says in the question that this man is stable; therefore you can assume that it is better to find out as much as you can before calling for help in this case. If the scenario was an emergency, however, you would call for help immediately.

D. *Searching through his mobile phone* is not an appropriate option, as you should not be using friends and family to get information about a patient unless it is a last resort. You should check the hospital database first.

E. *Starting the treatment anyway* is not a preferred option, as you should start investigations before management, **G** is therefore more suitable.

H. *Asking one of the nurses to try and track down some information* is not appropriate. Nurses are busy, and you are expected to take responsibility for finding patient information – or delegate it to the ward clerk if you are busy with the patient.

---

37. A 24-year-old woman is admitted to A&E following a paracetamol overdose. Her boyfriend brought her in when she admitted that she had taken 50 × 500 mg paracetamol tablets one hour earlier. Her boyfriend tells you she has been suffering from depression. You speak with her alone and she refuses any form of treatment – she wants to die. What *should* you do?

This is about recognising the need for senior help and tests your ability to handle patients who refuse to consent to treatment. Refer to Chapter 4 for more information on difficulties consenting patients.

C. *Bleeping the on-call psychiatrist* is appropriate, as you have information from her boyfriend that she has been suffering from depression. Moreover, this should be treated as an attempted suicide and therefore warrants psychiatric assessment. If you spoke to your registrar, they would advise you on a psychiatric referral. In this case you would need a rapid assessment on whether she has the capacity to refuse treatment.

B. *Seeing if the boyfriend can persuade her to change her mind* is appropriate. Using family and friends can be extremely helpful in getting patients to comply with treatment. Although this also puts him in a difficult situation, she may find it helpful talking to someone that she knows and has a close relationship with. You would still need to speak to psychiatry however.

D. *Calling your registrar* is appropriate, as this is not something that you would be expected to handle on your own as an FY1. You should call for senior help as soon as possible as this is a challenging situation.

E. *Treating her under the Mental Health Act (MHA)* is not a top selection, but is more appropriate than options **F** – *Treating her under the Mental Capacity Act (MCA)* – and **G** – *Treating her under the doctrine of necessity* – but you would

need a full assessment before jumping to commit her to treatment without consent. You would choose **E** over **F** as she doesn't meet the criteria for the MCA in that she understands that not having treatment will kill her. However, she is suffering from a mental health disorder and therefore can be treated against her will under the MHA. The situation of urgency is not so great that the doctrine of necessity (**G**) is warranted. Although this is an emergency, it is not such that you override the patient's wishes and act in their best interests anyway. She needs further assessment of her competence to refuse treatment.

A. *Respecting her right to refuse treatment* is not appropriate, as the history suggests that this patient's judgement may be compromised and therefore you should explore other options first.

H. *Discharging her from A&E* is not appropriate. You have a duty of care to this patient and dismissing her would question your professionalism.

---

38. You are working on a labour ward as an FY1. A nurse comes to see you to let you know that the ex-partner of one of the mothers is demanding to see his baby in the special care baby unit. He wasn't present at the birth and you know that the mother hasn't been in contact with him since she became pregnant. What *should* you do?

This is about patient confidentiality and protecting both the mother and the baby. This is also about recognising parental rights, and that you cannot refuse a parent access to a child just because of what the other parent says – providing, however, that you have confirmed identity.

C. *Asking the mother to confirm whether he is the father* is one of the most appropriate options, as you should seek consent from the mother whether to allow access to her baby – particularly as the father has been out of the picture for such a long time.

E. *Ringing the registrar to ask for advice* is appropriate, as you must consult a senior in tricky situations such as this. There could be potential problems from either the mother or this man, and you should alert seniors to this as soon as possible.

H. *Telling the man that he cannot see the baby until you have spoken to the mother* is one of the most appropriate options, as you must explain to him that the mother also has the right to know who will be visiting her child.

B. *Checking the baby's birth certificate* is not one of the preferred options, as you should always confirm whether the father is who he says he is. Another way would be to get the mother to confirm that he is the father.

A. *Taking this man to see the baby* is not appropriate, as – given the nature of their relationship – you should not allow the "alleged" father to see the baby without the mother's permission.

D. *Asking the midwife for advice* is not one of the preferred options as a nurse has come to you already asking for advice (rather than the midwife), suggesting that you are the most appropriate person to handle this situation.

F. *Documenting in the notes that this man wanted access to the baby* is also not one of the top selections; however, you would note this down at a later stage, as well as the conversation that you had with both parents.

G. *Telling the man to come back another time once he has pre-arranged a visit* is not one of the preferred options as fathers do not have to pre-arrange visits to see their children. Confirming his identity and getting consent is therefore more appropriate in this case.

---

39. A 79-year-old man is awaiting surgical repair of a fractured neck of femur. He tells you that he is a Jehovah's Witness and says he will refuse the operation if he needs a blood transfusion. You suspect the risk of needing a blood transfusion is high. He asks if there are any other options. What *should* you do?

> **ANSWER: AHF**

This question is about respecting a patient's wishes and acknowledging their rights to refuse treatment on the grounds of religious principles. See Chapter 4 for more information on Jehovah's Witnesses.

A. *Explaining the consequences of not having the operation* is appropriate. He should fully understand the risks of refusal. Moreover, there are conservative options but they are also risky.

H. *Finding out why he is opposed to a blood transfusion and his preferences* is also appropriate. You need to fully explore the patient's personal beliefs before deciding on a management plan. You can then relay this information to the registrar so that they are better informed of the patient's wishes.

F. *Bleeping your registrar to review the patient* is appropriate, as you always need senior advice in complex situations involving patient care. They will know whether there are cell-salvage facilities at your hospital, or whether he needs to be transferred to a different hospital. They can also enter into a more complex discussion with the patient regarding the relative risks and benefits of the various options available.

D. *Telling him you are unsure of the options but you will find out* is not a preferred option as your registrar must review the patient, in which case they can explain the options to him.

G. *Consulting your local guidelines* is also not a preferred option. Although there should be clear guidance on this at your local trust, this can be accessed after you have all the information from the patient and passed that on to the relevant senior. You would not want to delay this patient's treatment and therefore should act appropriately to make sure they receive senior review in a timely manner. Always be aware of where you can access such policies to read up at a later stage.

B. *Asking permission to contact the HLC* is not a top-ranked option. You need to gain consent before you can discuss his case with an external body. The HLC will be able to give you information on the options available to him, but this will take longer than getting an internal senior review where – knowing the options – it is likely that the HLC need not be contacted.

C. *Advising him to contact the Watchtower society* is not appropriate, as the patient does not have enough information to enquire about such a significant procedure at this stage. It is your responsibility to be an advocate for this patient and his care.

E. *Taking bloods and ordering pre-op investigations* is not appropriate, as the patient has not consented to the operation, and therefore these investigations are not considered a necessary part of their care.

---

40. A man is sitting in minors in A&E after having a drunken brawl with his friend. He has superficial lacerations to his shoulder and forearm. He arrived at midnight and, having been waiting for three hours, is getting increasingly agitated. The nurse comes to tell you that he is angry and threatening to self-discharge. You are busy packing the nose of his friend whom he was fighting with. What *should* you do?

> **ANSWER: BED**

This question is about staying calm whilst under pressure and maintaining a good relationship with patients through effective communication. See Chapter 4 for more information on verbal communication skills.

B. *Asking the nurse to let the patient know he is next* is the most appropriate response as it is clear he has been waiting a while and needs treatment.

E. *Telling the nurse to get the suture kit ready* is an appropriate response as this will help you out and save some time. It is important to recognise when it is appropriate to delegate tasks.

D. *Apologising to him for the long wait* is an appropriate response as this shows empathy. Hopefully this will diffuse his agitation and allow him to be treated. He could very well be agitated because he is in pain or he doesn't like hospitals. It is important not to label patients as "difficult" or "drunk" as this could impair your responsibility to treat them in their best interests.

A. *Allowing him to self-discharge* is not appropriate, as you have a duty of care to your patients. There is no indication that this patient is going to physically abuse the nurse, or that the nurse feels threatened in any way. Therefore it is best if they are persuaded to stay and receive treatment.

C. *Calling security* is not appropriate at this stage, as he is not being threatening towards staff or others; he is merely saying that he will discharge himself against medical advice.

F. *Asking the nurse to tell him he should wait because you are seeing his friend* is not appropriate, as it is better to let him know he is next (B). Although he may be aware that his friend is also in hospital, this could still be considered a breach of confidentiality. It is better to keep information as anonymous as possible.

G. *Leaving his friend and going to attend to his shoulder and forearm lacerations* is not appropriate, as you should finish treating one patient rather than abandoning them to attend to another patient.

H. *Calling the SHO to review and suture him* is not appropriate. You should be able to manage this situation as an FY1. You should avoid calling the SHO for minor disagreements that you are more than capable of handling. However, if this was a laceration to the forehead, you might be concerned that the increasing agitation was a manifestation of a more serious head injury, in which case you would consider bleeping the SHO for a full head injury assessment.

---

41. You are in the surgical assessment unit and trying to consent a 55-year-old man for rigid sigmoidoscopy that you will be doing under supervision. You have been trained to consent for this procedure and are aware of all the risks and benefits. When you try to explain the procedure, he says "Do whatever you think is best, Doc, I don't want to know". What *should* you do?

This is about handling a situation where a patient does not wish to consent to treatment. See Chapter 3 for more information on consent in patients with capacity.

C. *Telling him it is important that he understands the procedure in order to consent* is appropriate, as you should reiterate the need for an explanation of the procedure. The patient may still change his mind about knowing.

A. *Telling him you need to give him a brief explanation of the procedure* is appropriate, as you must be honest with your patient and reason with him as to why he should be involved in his care. Patients should know the broad nature of the procedure, as it is possible to proceed without providing all the information on the risks and benefits.

E. *Asking him whether he would prefer to have a family member with him* is appropriate. Even though this man has to consent to the procedure himself, many patients prefer to have a relative present. The added benefit of having a relative is that they are likely to take on board more information than the patient and can ask questions that the patient otherwise wouldn't. This is a way of indirectly engaging the patient in a conversation about the procedure beyond the brief explanation given to him and may encourage the patient to ask questions himself.

D. *Phoning your registrar to consent the patient* is not a preferred option. You have all the knowledge that the senior has to consent this patient. Moreover, as you will be doing the procedure yourself (under supervision), it would be more appropriate for you to gain the consent. You should try persuading the patient first, before seeking senior help.

B. *Asking him to sign the form without going into detail* is not appropriate, as this is not getting appropriate consent – selecting this option would question your probity and integrity

F. *Explaining the procedure to a family member instead* is not appropriate, as a family member cannot consent for a patient with capacity and can only do so in a patient who lacks capacity if they are named as a legal proxy.

G. *Cancelling the investigation* is not appropriate, as this response is premature. You should try alternatives before jumping to cancel an investigation that is designed to help the patient – a senior would be expected to make this decision.

H. *Filling in the form yourself and signing in his best interests* is not appropriate – this is breaking the professional code of conduct and questions your honesty and professionalism.

---

42. You are looking after Mrs Chang who is intermittently confused. Her family are all in the waiting room and are anxious to know how Mrs Chang is doing. You have the results of her CT scan which is normal. What *should* you do?

This is about ensuring patient confidentiality in a patient who may or may not have the capacity to consent. It is also about strengthening relationships with relatives and maintaining good communication.

B. *Going to see how Mrs Chang is today* is appropriate, as you should determine whether she has capacity or not. As she is intermittently confused, you should wait to tell her the news until she can comprehend it. Telling the family before the patient is never acceptable – unless you are sure that she is never going to have capacity.

D. *Telling her family about her general well-being without going into specific details* is appropriate. The family will want to know how she is today and it is important that family members are kept up to date with her clinical situation. If you explain that you have to get consent from the patient they should understand and will appreciate that you have addressed their anxieties.

H. *Ringing the registrar to ask for advice* is appropriate, as you have a duty to relay results to patients in a timely manner. You will need advice on this matter as it is likely that the family are worried and will ask you about this. Confidentiality and consent are complex issues which often extend beyond what you can see. In this respect, it is always a good idea to get a senior involved early rather than having to undo a mistake later.

G. *Viewing the scan yourself* is not a preferred option. Although it is good practice to look at all scans as well as the radiology report, Mrs Chang and her family should take priority. Viewing normal CT scans is just as important as viewing abnormal ones and this is a learning opportunity, but, ideally, you would need a senior to talk you through the scan to consolidate information accurately.

F. *Letting your colleagues know Mrs Chang's result* is not a preferred option. You should let your colleagues know the results at handover or a more appropriate time. The priority here is to ascertain how you are going to get the results to Mrs Chang.

E. *Waiting until Mrs Chang asks specifically for her results* is not a top selection because you should actively seek to speak to relatives when results are available – provided you have the consent from the patient to do so.

A. *Telling the family the good news* and **C** *Asking a nurse to tell the family the good news* are not appropriate, as the patient has a right to know their results before the family, regardless of who delivers the news.

---

43. **You are working on an oncology ward. You are sitting at the desk ordering bloods when your colleague Jane tells you she thinks that you are not picking up your fair share of work. You feel Jane is boisterous and arrogant. No one else has mentioned anything to you about being lazy and you feel you are competent. What *should* you do?**

> **ANSWER: CED**

This is about managing interpersonal relationships and conflict within a team. You are expected to maintain harmony and work effectively as a team-player. Refer to Chapter 6 for more information on teamwork.

C. *Saying you cannot discuss this here and suggesting a more appropriate place* is a top selection, as you never want to get into an argument on the ward in front of patients. This would be unprofessional.

E. *Asking Jane why she feels you are not doing your share* is appropriate, as you should find out from your colleague why she has a problem with you. That way you can discuss it openly and hopefully reach a compromise.

D. *Suggesting that you divide the jobs evenly* is appropriate, as this means that neither of you can complain about the workload. Resolving the problem between you is far more appropriate than involving seniors. You are adults and should be able to work through this.

H. *Reporting the bullying to your consultant* and **F** *Raising the issue with your educational supervisor* are not appropriate, as you should not escalate things at this stage. Try to resolve the conflict amongst yourselves.

A. *Telling Jane you think she is arrogant* and **B** *Arguing that you do your fair share* are not appropriate, as neither response is constructive and will likely lead to more arguments rather than a solution.

G. *Asking your other colleagues their opinion of you* is not appropriate, as involving team members may mean asking colleagues to take sides. You are expected to maintain harmony within the team as far as possible.

---

44. **You are working on a busy respiratory ward. One of your colleagues, Jack, is consistently lazy to the point where he may be compromising patient care. The nurses and ward** cover at handover have commented on this. What *should* you do?

> **ANSWER: BEG**

This question is also about teamwork and knowing how to handle a struggling colleague.

B. *Asking Jack whether he feels he is struggling* is appropriate, as you should find out whether your colleague feels there is a problem. You can then engage in a conversation as to whether Jack has insight into his behaviour, whether he feels he is struggling, or whether he is just attempting to get out of his share of the work.

E. *Recommending the nurse in charge has a quiet word* is as appropriate. Given that the nurses have commented on Jack's behaviour, it would be appropriate for them to intervene. Working as part of a multi-disciplinary team, the nurse in charge should feel they have authority to speak to an FY1 if they are concerned about their behaviour.

G. *Informing your consultant that Jack is struggling* is appropriate. Whilst it is courteous to share this information with your colleague before your consultant, the question suggests that patient care is being compromised. Hence, your consultant needs to be informed of the situation. Moreover, given a few members of the team have commented, it is right to escalate this further. If you did nothing, you would be letting down your colleagues, Jack and the patients under his care.

C. *Telling Jack that he is not doing his share of the workload* is not as appropriate. Highlighting your awareness of the situation to your colleague may produce very little gain in terms of resolving the problem. Moreover, it may be better that this information comes from the nurse in charge who has expressed a concern.

H. *Telling Jack you will speak to your educational supervisor if things don't change* is not a preferred option as your educational supervisor is only in a position to give you advice and, unless they happen to be Jack's educational supervisor too, cannot help him in the same way that his own educational supervisor should.

A. *Offering to take on some of Jack's workload* is not appropriate. This would increase pressure on you, in an already busy situation. Moreover, this is not addressing the real issue. You could always help them out if you have finished your jobs, but, ideally, they need to seek help from their educational supervisor if they cannot cope.

D. *Informing the foundation programme clinical lead* is not appropriate, as there are more suitable reporting channels.

F. *Asking the nurses to fill in a CAE form* is not appropriate, as you should speak Jack before filling in a CAE form regarding his conduct. This would also be escalated outside the team and Jack would be referred to see the foundation programme clinical lead. There is no indication in the question of one specific incident compromising care that would require filling in this form.

45. You send a medical student to take some bloods; for which they are trained. You check the results at 3 p.m. and realise that the samples are all coagulated. What *should* you do?

ANSWER: AEG

This question is about teaching medical students to take responsibility for their own actions and own up to mistakes.

A. *Retaking the bloods* is appropriate, as the patient comes first, and the mistake must be corrected.

E. *Supervising the student when taking bloods next time* is appropriate, as the question indicates an issue with the samples taken. It would be helpful for you to go with the student to ensure they are doing the job correctly and to give them practical advice. You can also take this opportunity to discuss with them the difficulties associated with venepuncture.

G. *Suggesting the student reflects on this incident in their portfolio* is appropriate. Reflecting means the student can learn about the consequences of not checking what they have done is right, and the implications for the patient. This will be an important learning point for the student which they should not ignore.

C. *Pointing out the mistake to the student* is not a preferred option. Although you are responsible for teaching and learning, it would be better to supervise them where a problem has occurred rather than highlighting the error and moving on.

F. *Telling the student to bring the sample to you next time* is also not a top selection, as it would be better to supervise the student rather than just checking that the bloods are OK before sending them to the laboratory. It is good practice to check them regardless – especially if it is for something like a blood transfusion.

B. *Reporting the student to your consultant* is not appropriate, as this puts the student in an awkward position and you don't want to scare them away from attempting venepuncture ever again.

D. *Ignoring their mistake is not appropriate*, as the student will not learn if it is ignored.

H. *Telling the student to get some more clinical skills training before they go onto the wards* is not appropriate, as the best practice involves real patients. They have already been trained in venepuncture and telling them to go back to square one will dent their confidence further. You should be supportive towards students to most effectively enable their learning.

46. You are working in a GP's surgery. A patient comes in to see you with symptoms of angina at rest. It says on the system that the GP told them last time not to drive. You ask them whether they have been driving, and they tell you they have: they drove to the surgery today. What *should* you do?

ANSWER: ECG

This question tests your knowledge of effective communication concerning patient guidance. See Chapter 2 for more information on the DVLA.

E. *Asking if they remember the GP advising them not to drive* is appropriate, as you should reiterate that you know they have been given this information already. This is more polite than option **F**.

C. *Advising them to stop driving until their symptoms are under control* is appropriate, as you should relay the advice they have already received about not driving with symptoms of angina.

G. *Consulting the GP for advice* is appropriate. Although you should be aware of the guidance and can give patient the appropriate advice (**C**), this is a tricky situation and you should seek senior help on how to proceed.

D. *Finding out whether someone can drive them home* is not a preferred option as you should find out from the GP how best to proceed with getting the patient home. This would, however, establish whether someone could come and collect them to drive them home.

A. *Reporting them to the DVLA* is not appropriate, as you should not inform the DVLA without the patient's consent. Also, it is the patient's responsibility to do this, if necessary.

B. *Advising them to inform the DVLA* is not appropriate, as it may be that the patient misinterpreted the advice given by the GP. Also, the DVLA guidance suggests that driving must cease until symptoms are under control but they need not be notified for angina.

F. *Reminding them that last time the GP asked them not to drive* is not a preferred option as it is more aggressive than E and the patient may have forgotten they were asked not to drive.

H. *Asking them to hand over their keys* is not appropriate, as, once their symptoms are adequately controlled, they should be allowed to drive. It would be advisable for someone to pick them up, but if you are so worried you have to confiscate their keys – they probably should be going to hospital rather than home.

47. Your consultant on a ward round orders a spine MRI and asks you to put in the request. You overhear the registrar saying to another colleague that it is not indicated. What *should* you do?

ANSWER: BEF

This question is about managing conflicts within a team and maintaining harmony whilst making sure the more appropriate action is taken.

B. *Asking the consultant the reasons for ordering the MRI* is appropriate, as this could simply be an opportunity for learning about indications for a particular scan. Moreover, you should be putting this on the request form.

E. *Asking the registrar why they think the MRI is not indicated* is appropriate, as this would be an opportunity for conflict resolution. If you find out the reasons that the registrar disagrees with the indication, you can explain clearly why the consultant ordered the MRI.

F. *Ringing the radiologist to discuss the MRI request* is appropriate. Radiologists are busy, but they would appreciate you politely ringing to discuss an MRI request. Moreover, you can include any indications you discuss on the form which will help the radiographer select the best images. The radiologist could also raise concerns if they felt that the scan wasn't indicated, in which case you could relay that information back to your consultant.

A. *Ordering the MRI as the consultant has requested* is not appropriate. Although you should never undermine your consultant, you cannot ignore the comments of your registrar. Patient care should come before disagreements, and patients should only have scans when indicated.

C. *Ignoring the consultant and following your registrar* is rarely appropriate, if ever. You should not ignore your consultant or go against their decision without their knowledge. In the event there was a change to their management plan and they could not be contacted, you would have to document everything in the notes including the arguments on both sides and why the final decision was made. Under no circumstances should you deliberately undermine your consultant.

D. *Telling the consultant that the registrar does not think the MRI is indicated* is not appropriate, as you have a duty not to create conflict within your team.

H. *Documenting in the notes that the MRI was ordered but that the registrar disagreed* is not a preferred option. Ideally you should not document disagreements within the team in the notes – unless they are directly relevant to patient safety.

---

48. You are working as an FY1 as part of the medical on-call team. A patient with type I diabetes came in with diabetic ketoacidosis (DKA), but is improving having been on a sliding-scale. The consultant prescribes short-acting insulin. The patient disagrees with this and asks that he be put back onto his regular insulin regimen of long-acting insulin. What *should* you do?

ANSWER: AGB

This question is about advocating for your patient and utilising expert knowledge within your team.

A. *Asking the specialist diabetic nurse for advice* is appropriate, as they have a wealth of knowledge regarding the prescribing of insulin and, if needs be, can act as another advocate for the patient using their expertise.

G. *Asking the patient why they don't want to have short-acting insulin* is appropriate, as you want to find out the patient's wishes before you can discuss them with the senior in charge.

B. *Calling the consultant to relay the patient's disapproval of their regimen* is also appropriate, as you must – at all times – be an advocate for your patient and meet their wishes as far as possible. If a patient is unhappy with their care, you have a duty to let your consultant know about it – tactfully!

C. *Prescribing long-acting insulin* **D** *Telling the patient they are on the right insulin* and **H** *Ignoring the patient's request* are not appropriate, as these options all ignore the patient's wishes and their rights to be involved in treatment.

E. *Telling the patient they will have to discuss the option with the consultant* is not appropriate, as this postpones the issue and it is your job to broach the subject with the consultant, not theirs.

F. *Writing both up on the drug chart to be delivered* is not appropriate, as this leaves potential for a prescribing error if it is not clear which insulin should be delivered to the patient and when.

---

49. A 69-year-old man is brought into A&E with symptoms later confirmed as an ischaemic stroke. Your specialist registrar reviews him in A&E and writes up his prescription on a drug chart. The patient reaches you on the stroke ward one hour later with his notes and a different drug chart. Clopidogrel is written up STAT but not given. The prescription written is not the one that your registrar wrote. What *should* you do?

ANSWER: BCG

This is about recognising the potential for a prescribing error which could potentially harm the patient. Remember not to PANIC when prescribing: Prescription, Allergy, Notes, Interactions, Clear. This error involves the prescription, i.e. ensuring that only one dose of the medication is given (where 85% of errors occur), and the notes i.e. two drug charts. See Chapter 3 for more details.

B. *Bleeping your registrar* is appropriate, as you need to find out what happened to the other drug chart and whether the patient has received their Clopidogrel.

C. *Taking the chart down to A&E whilst looking for the other one* is appropriate, as you can ask the nurses where this patient was and whether they know anything about the prescription as well as having a look for the drug chart. This should quickly resolve the situation and, as a matter of urgency, should be your responsibility.

G. *Delaying giving the Clopidogrel until the other chart is found* is appropriate. Although nearly all patients receive anticoagulation in hospital for deep vein thrombosis (DVT) prophylaxis, you would not want to put them at risk of an intracranial bleed by titrating them outside of the therapeutic range. Given this patient has had an ischaemic stroke, this situation does need to be resolved promptly, but delaying is the safer option.

A. *Ringing the pharmacy to ask for advice* is not appropriate. It is unlikely that pharmacy will be able to give you any indication of whether the patient has received the Clopidogrel or not. They can provide advice on the correct protocol – but these options are available. This question tests your knowledge of safe practice.

D. *Asking the patient whether they have been given the Clopidogrel* is not appropriate, as the patient may not have an idea of what they have been given and you could be given false information. It is best to rely on the facts – which means finding both charts.

E. *Giving the Clopidogrel* and **F** *Giving half the dose of Clopidogrel* are not appropriate, as they both put the patient at risk of bleeding. Medication should not be changed or given without having all the accurate and relevant information.

H. *Telling the nurses not to give Clopidogrel to the patient* is not a preferred option. Although communication is key to preventing errors, the nurses would not give the prescription without seeing the chart (nor if you crossed it out). If you take the chart down with you to A&E, this will prevent the patient receiving the medication.

---

50. You are working on a busy cardiology ward. Your colleague is on call and asks you to hold their bleep for them whilst they go and get some lunch. What *should* you do?

This question is about trying to help out your colleague but recognising that it is not appropriate to pass over your bleep.
C. *Politely declining because you have your own patients* is appropriate, as you should not take someone else's bleep when you are not on-call. You have a responsibility for your own patients and they have to be your priority. Taking on another workload on an already busy ward is not acceptable.
E. *Seeing if they have any outstanding jobs you can help with* is appropriate, as this is offering your colleague support so they can find some time to go and get their lunch. That way you stay on the ward without taking on any new patients.
F. *Offering to get their lunch for them* is appropriate, as this will be helping out your colleague by saving them time so they can take a shorter break to sit down and eat it.
A. *Agreeing to hold their bleep* is not appropriate. You should not hold someone else's bleep – unless under exceptional circumstances such as breaking bad news.

B. *Offering to go with them for their lunch* is not appropriate. If you want to help your colleague out, you should stay on the ward and go for your own lunch when you get an opportunity.
D. *Suggesting they get in touch with someone from the on-call team to hold their bleep* is not appropriate. You should not give your bleep to anyone else. More importantly, if your colleague is busy, the other members of the on-call team are also likely to be busy.
G. *Telling them to turn it off whilst they go and get some lunch* is not appropriate. There might be a sick patient whom your colleague needs to attend to, and therefore not being accessible could compromise patient care.
H. *Suggesting they go quickly to get their lunch* is not appropriate, as this does not help out your colleague.

Beyond this book

Try to expand on your experiences with scenarios. Box 8.1 includes a list of useful questions for you to ask your FY1 colleagues whilst on clinical placements as well as some tasks for you to observe.

Finally, Box 8.2 is designed to show you how you can build your own examples on the wards. Comment on the area you feel the situation most accurately highlights and then describe the situation and why there was a problem. You should then analyse how that situation played out and consider it against the best practice material that is outlined in this book. At the end of this exercise you should reflect on your learning as that way you will cement the example well and truly for the future!

One final bit of advice to remember is, "It is a really stressful job at times but it's really good fun" – Nick FY1.

Box 8.1 Useful Questions

Commitment to professionalism:
• Where have you seen confidentiality being compromised?
• Have you ever had to challenge inappropriate behaviour?
• Ask about the teaching available and find out how they juggle their priorities.

Coping with pressure:
• What pressures do you find yourself under?
• Have you ever made a mistake? What did you do about it?
• Have you ever experienced a confrontational situation?
• Who do you turn to when you need help?

Effective communication:
• Go with a doctor to see how they negotiate a scan for radiology.
• Go with a doctor to see a death certificate/cremation form being filled in.
• Listen to a referral and practise the SBAR approach.

Patient focus:
• Observe times where patient concerns and views are integrated into management.
• Observe the options given to patients about their treatment. What did you learn about their needs and were they adequately addressed?

Team working:
• Have you ever had difficulties with a colleague? What were they?
• Offer assistance to the juniors on the ward and ask them how they prioritise their jobs on a daily basis.
• Speak to other healthcare professionals about their roles and responsibilities.

Box 8.2 Build your own scenario

Judgement area: Commitment to professionalism

Situation: Doctor was needed on the ward but also had teaching scheduled.

Dilemma: Patient care comes first, but doctors are also responsible for their own learning. How urgent are the tasks on the ward? How essential is it that they attend the teaching? Can they rely on their colleagues to get the relevant information for them if they cannot get away?

What the doctor did: Got very stressed about the fact that they had to be two places at once.

What the doctor should have done: Analysed the dilemma calmly and weighed the positives and negatives of going to teaching or not before acting on their decision. The doctor decided to stay on the ward and asked a colleague to make notes for them as otherwise they would be delayed at work for too long.

Reflection: I learned that you should always try to meet your commitment to attend teaching, but that patient care comes first; hence, there may be times where you have to compromise and sacrifice your own learning.

AMRC (Academy of Medical Royal Colleges) (2010) *ST1 Selection Pilot 2010: Project Report*. London: UCL.

Baille, W.F., Buckman, R. and Lenzi, R. (2000) SPIKES – a six-step protocol for delivering bad news: application to the patient with cancer. *The Oncologist*, **5**(4): 302–311.

Belbin, M.R. (2008) *The Belbin Guide to Succeeding at Work* (2nd ed.). Cambridge: Belbin Associates.

Belbin, M.R. (2010a [1981]) *Management Teams. Why They Succeed or Fail* (3rd ed.). Oxford: Butterworth-Heinemann.

Belbin, M.R. (2010b [1993]) *Team Roles at Work* (2nd ed.). Oxford: Butterworth-Heinemann.

BMA (British Medical Association) (2004a) *Communication Skills Education for Doctors: An Update*. London: BMA. Also available at: http://faculty.ksu.edu.sa/nadalyousefi/communication%20skills/Communication%20skills.pdf (accessed 7 August 2012).

BMA (British Medical Association) (2004b) *Safe Handover: Safe Patients. Guidance on Clinical Handover for Clinicians and Managers*. London, BMA. Also available at: http://bma.org.uk/-/media/Files/PDFs/Practical%20advice%20at%20work/Contracts/safe%20handover%20safe%20patients.pdf (accessed 11 August 2012).

BMA (British Medical Association) (2011) *Using Social Media: Practical and Ethical Guidance for Doctors and Medical Students*. Available at: http://www.medschools.ac.uk/SiteCollectionDocuments/social_media_guidance_may2011.pdf (accessed 11 August 2012).

BPS (British Pharmacological Society) (2010) *Ten Principles of Good Prescribing*. Available at: http://main.bps.ac.uk/SpringboardWebApp/userfiles/bps/file/Guidelines/BPSPrescribingPrinciples.pdf (accessed 6 August 2012).

Covey, S. (2004) *The Seven Habits of Highly Effective People* (2nd edition). London: Simon and Schuster.

Crocker, C., Kapila, R., Carney, A. et al. (2010) *Improving Patient Safety: SBAR*. University of Nottingham [elearning tool]. Available at: http://www.nottingham.ac.uk/nmp/sonet/rlos/patientsafety/sbar/ (accessed 6 August 2012).

DCA (Department for Constitutional Affairs) (2005) *Mental Capacity Act: Code of Practice* (section 3.6). London: The Stationery Office.

DH (Department of Health) (2000) *An Organisation with a Memory*. London: The Stationery Office.

DH (Department of Health) (2001), *Building a safer NHS for patients*. London: The Stationery Office.

Department of Health (2010) *The Caldicott Guardian Manual 2010*. London: Department of Health. Also available at: http://www.dh.gov.uk/en/Publicationsandstatistics/Publications/PublicationsPolicyAndGuidance/DH_114509 (accessed 11 August 2012).

Directgov (2011) *Communication Support for Deaf People*. Available at: http://www.direct.gov.uk/en/disabledpeople/everydaylifeandaccess/everydayaccess/dg_10037996 (accessed 7 August 2012).

Directgov (2012) *Disabled people*. Available at: http://www.direct.gov.uk/en/DisabledPeople/index.htm (accessed 7 August 2012).

Disability Discrimination Act (DDA) (1995) *Disability Discrimination Act 1995*. London: HMSO. Also available at: http://www.legislation.gov.uk/ukpga/1995/50/contents (accessed 7 August 2012).

DVLA (Driver and Vehicle Licensing Agency) (2011) *At a Glance Guide to the Current Medical Standards of Fitness to Drive*. Swansea: Drivers Medical Group.

EHRC (Equality and Human Rights Commission) (2010) *Good Medical Practice and Disability Equality*. Available at: http://www.equalityhumanrights.com/advice-and-guidance/before-the-equality-act/guidance-for-service-providers-pre-october-2010/good-medical-practice-and-disability-equality/ (accessed 11 December 2011).

GMC (General Medical Council) (2006) *The Meaning of Fitness to Practise*. Available at http://www.gmc-uk.org/the_meaning_of_fitness_to_practise.pdf_25416562.pdf (accessed 12 August 2012).

GMC (General Medical Council) (2008a) *Consent Guidance: Patients and Doctors Making Decisions Together*. London: GMC. Also available at: http://www.gmc-uk.org/guidance/ethical_guidance/consent_guidance_index.asp (accessed 12 August 2012).

GMC (General Medical Council) (2008b) *Personal Beliefs and Medical Practice: Supplementary Guidance*. London: GMC. Also available at: http://www.gmc-uk.org/static/documents/content/Personal_Beliefs.pdf (accessed 7 August 2012).

GMC (General Medical Council) (2008c) *Raising Concerns about Patient Safety*. Available at: http://www.gmc-uk.org/static/documents/content/Raising_concerns.pdf (accessed 7 August 2012).

GMC (General Medical Council) (2009a) *Good Medical Practice*. Available at: http://www.gmc-uk.org/guidance/good_medical_practice.asp (accessed 11 August 2012).

GMC (General Medical Council) (2009b) *Confidentiality: Reporting Concerns about Patients to the DVLA or the DVA*. Available at http://www.gmc-uk.org/Confidentiality_reporting_concerns_DVLA_2009.pdf_27494214.pdf (accessed 8 August 2012).

GMC (General Medical Council) (2009c) *Confidentiality: Reporting Gunshot and Knife Wounds*. Available at: http://www.gmc-uk.org/Confidentiality_reporting_gunshot_wounds_2009.pdf_27493825.pdf (accessed 8 August 2012).

GMC (General Medical Council) (2009d) *Confidentiality*. Available at: http://www.gmc-uk.org/Confidentiality___English_0910.pdf_48902982.pdf (accessed 8 August 2012).

The Situational Judgement Test at a Glance, First Edition. Frances Varian and Lara Cartwright.

88 © 2013 John Wiley & Sons, Ltd. Published 2013 by John Wiley & Sons, Ltd.

GMC (General Medical Council) (2009e) *0–18 Years Guidance for All Doctors*. London: GMC. Also available at: http://www.gmc-uk.org/guidance/ethical_guidance/children_guidance_index.asp (accessed 11 August 2012).

GMC (General Medical Council) (2009f) *Confidentiality: Disclosing Information about Serious Communicable Diseases*. Available at: http://www.gmc-uk.org/Confidentiality_disclosing_info_serious_commun_diseases_2009.pdf_27493404.pdf (accessed 12 August 2012).

GMC (General Medical Council) (2010) *Treatment and Care towards End of Life: Good Practice in Decision-Making*. London: GMC. Also available at: http://www.gmc-uk.org/End_of_life.pdf_32486688.pdf (accessed 12 August 2012).

GMC (General Medical Council) (2011a: 28) *0–18 years guidance for all doctors*. London: GMC. Also available at: http://www.gmc-uk.org/guidance/ethical_guidance/children_guidance_index.asp (accessed 18 August 2012).

GMC (General Medical Council) (2011b: para 60) *0–18 years guidance for all doctors*. London: GMC. Also available at: http://www.gmc-uk.org/guidance/ethical_guidance/children_guidance_index.asp (accessed 18 August 2012).

GMC (General Medical Council) (2012) *Raising and acting on concerns about patient safety*. Manchester: GMC. Also available at: http://www.gmc-uk.org/guidance/ethical_guidance/raising_concerns.asp (accessed 7 August 2012).

Howard, R., Avery, A.J., Slavenburg, S. et al. (2007) Which drugs cause preventable admissions to hospital? A systematic review. *British Journal of Clinical Pharmacology* **63**(2): 136–147.

ISFP (Improving Selection to Foundation programme) (2012) website. Available at http://www.isfp.org.uk/Pages/default.aspx [accessed March 2012].

Kurtz, S.M. (1989) Curriculum structuring to enhance communication skills development. In M. Stewart and D. Roter (eds), *Communication with Medical Patients*. Newbury Park, CA: Sage Publications.

Lee, S. (2007) *Making Decisions: The Independent Mental Capacity Advocate (IMCA) Service*. London: Mental Capacity Implementation Programme.

Lesar, T.S., Briceland, L., and Stein, D.S. (1997) Factors related to errors in medication prescribing. *Journal of the American Medical Association* **277**: 312–317.

Maxwell, S. and Walley, T. (2003) Teaching safe and effective prescribing in UK medical schools: a core curriculum for tomorrow's doctors. *British Journal of Clinical Pharmacology* **55**(6): 496–503.

Myers and Briggs Foundation (n.d.) MBTI Basics. Available at: http://www.myersbriggs.org/my-mbti-personality-type/mbti-basics/ (accessed 6 August 2012).

MCA (Mental Capacity Act) (2005) *Act of Parliament UK*; available from: http://www.legislation.gov.uk/ukpga/2005/9/contents.

McCrae, R.R., Terracciano, A. et al. (2005). Universal features of personality traits from the observer's perspective: data from 50 different cultures. *Journal of Personality and Social Psychology*; **88**: 547–561.

MHRA (Medicines and Healthcare products Regulatory Agency) (2012) MHRA website. Available at: http://www.mhra.gov.uk/#page=DynamicListMedicines (accessed 9 August 2012).

MPS (Medical Protection Society) (2010) *GP Trainee: Confidentiality*. Available at: http://www.medicalprotection.org/Default.aspx?DN=0d676448-316d-46d7-b1c3-ac34b3ff4c8a (accessed 9 August 2012).

MPS (Medical Protection Society) (2011) *Avoiding Easy Mistakes: Five Medicolegal Hazards for Interns and SHOs*. London: MPS. Also available at: http://www.medicalprotection.org/ireland/booklets/medicolegal-hazards (accessed 9 August 2012).

Ministry of Ethics (2010) *Consent and Confidentiality*. Available at: http://ministryofethics.co.uk/index.php?p=6 (accessed 8 August 2012).

Ministry of Justice (2012) *The Cremation (England and Wales) Regulations 2008: Guidance to Medical Practitioners Completing Forms Cremation 4 and 5*. [pdf]

NICE (2011) *Caesarean Section*. London: NICE. Also available at: http://guidance.nice.org.uk/cg132 (accessed 12 August 2012).

ODI (Office for Disability Issues) (2010) *Equality Act: Guidance on Matters to be Taken into Account in Determining Questions Relating to the Definition of Disability* (A1. A3. C1). London: ODI.

ONS (The Office of National Statistics) (2010) *Guidance for Doctors Completing Medical Certificates or Cause of Death in England and Wales*. Available at: http://www.kentlmc.org/kentlmc/website10.nsf/0/61a64422c4e7aa1b80257a38003f6bf1/$FILE/medcert_July_2010.pdf (accessed 7 August 2012).

PALS (Patient Advice and Liaison Service) (2009) What is PALS? Available at: http://www.pals.nhs.uk/cmsContentView.aspx?ItemID=932 (accessed 7 August 2012).

Patel, V. and Morrissey, J. (2011) *Practical and Professional Clinical Skills*. Oxford: Oxford University Press.

Patterson, F., Archer, V., Kerrin, M. et al. (2010) Appendix D: FY1 Job Analysis. In Medical Schools Council, *Improving Selection to Foundation Programme Final Report*. Work Psychology Group and University of Cambridge, pp 126–240. Available at: http://www.medschools.ac.uk/SiteCollectionDocuments/Final%20Report%20of%20ISFP%20Project%20Group.pdf (accessed 7 August 2012).

Phelan, M. and Parkman, S. (1995) How to work with an interpreter. *British Medical Journal* **311**: 555–557.

Rosen, S. and Tesser, A. (1970). On reluctance to communicate undesirable information: the MUM effect. *Sociometry* **33**(3): 253–263.

RCS (The Royal College of Surgeons of England) (2007) *Safe Handover: Guidance from the Working Time Directive working party*. Available at: http://www.rcseng.ac.uk/publications/docs/publication.2007-05-14.3777986999/ (accessed 12 August 2012).

Scottish Government (2009) *Guidance for Medical Staff Completing Medical Certificates of the Cause of Death*. Available at: http://www.sehd.scot.nhs.uk/cmo/CMO(2009)10.pdf (accessed 12 August 2012).

Index